OXFORD MEDICAL PUBLICATIONS

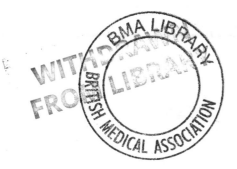

Oxford Core Texts

Clinical Dermatology
Clinical Skills
Endocrinology
Health and Illness in the Community
Human Physiology
Medical Genetics
Medical Imaging
Neurology
Oncology
Palliative Care
Psychiatry

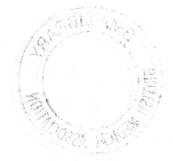

Neurology

SECOND EDITION

Michael Donaghy

Reader in Clinical Neurology, University of Oxford,
Consultant Neurologist, Radcliffe Infirmary, Oxford

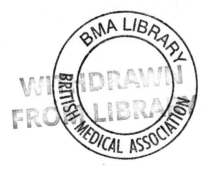

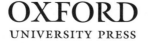

OXFORD
UNIVERSITY PRESS

OXFORD
UNIVERSITY PRESS

Great Clarendon Street, Oxford OX2 6DP

Oxford University Press is a department of the University of Oxford.
It furthers the University's objective of excellence in research, scholarship,
and education by publishing worldwide in

Oxford New York

Auckland Bangkok Buenos Aires Cape Town Chennai
Dar es Salaam Delhi Hong Kong Istanbul Karachi Kolkata
Kuala Lumpur Madrid Melbourne Mexico City Mumbai Nairobi
São Paulo Shanghai Taipei Tokyo Toronto

Oxford is a registered trade mark of Oxford University Press
in the UK and in certain other countries

Published in the United States
by Oxford University Press Inc., New York

A catalogue record for the this title is available from the British Library

Library of Congress Cataloguing in Publication Data attached

Neurology / Michael Donaghy. 2nd edn. (Oxford Medical Publication. (Oxford Core Texts).

Includes bibliographical references and index.
1. Neurology. I. Title. II. Series. III. Series: Oxford core texts.
[DNLM: 1. Nervous System Diseases–diagnosis. 2. Medical History Taking–methods.
3. Neurologic Examination–methods. WL 141 D674n 2005]
RC 346. D66 2005   616.8–dc22   2004019158
ISBN 0 19 852636 9 (Pbk: alk paper)

10 9 8 7 6 5 4 3 2 1

Typeset by EXPO Holdings Sdn Bhd., Malaysia
Printed in GreatBritain
on acid-free paper by Ashford Colour Press Ltd., Gosport, Hampshire

Preface to the second edition

As before, this new edition aims to provide students with a sound clinical approach to the common problems encountered in neurological practice, and to teach pertinent neurological examination. The text has been revised throughout, and introduces new developments in everyday practice. New material includes chapters on somatosensory abnormalities, autonomic abnormalities, and gait disorders and falls.

The main innovation is the inclusion of 24 case histories at the end of chapters. The discussion following each case should be regarded as an integral part of the text. They show how the foregoing general principles of neurology can be applied to the practical problems posed by individual patients and the fascination of how neurological diseases interface with everyday life. Some highlight diseases, or clinical approaches, that are not covered in the main text. Some cases introduce important new treatments such as botulinum toxin injections, intravenous immunoglobulin, and interventional radiology. They are not intended as self-assessment exercises.

I remain extremely grateful to all those who helped prepare the first edition; their work laid the foundations for this revision. Joanna Wilkinson has prepared the new text with a deft mixture of patience and alacrity. Valuable advice about the statistical presentation of treatment benefits was provided by P. Rothwell. There are many new figures for which I am grateful to P. Anslow, A. Molyneux, L. Percy, and N. White. Once again, I must thank the staff of Oxford University Press for encouraging this second edition, and their skilful work on its production.

Oxford, July 2004   Michael Donaghy

Preface to the first edition

Many students and doctors regard neurology as being forbiddingly difficult. The huge range of diseases, many of them rare, makes it hard to sift out the common clinical problems. The neurological examination is often seen as excessively lengthy, hard to master, and even harder to interpret. And yet, when students watch a modern-day neurologist at work in outpatients, they realize that fewer than a dozen clinical problems account for three-quarters of the consultations, and that usually a neurologist can examine the patient within two or three minutes.

The central purpose of this book is to give students a working knowledge of the common clinical problems in neurology, and to teach a simple, quick, and reliable neurological examination. The book does not provide a traditional account of neurological diseases, classified according to the pathological process. Rather, it takes clinical problems as a framework for discussing the important diseases, and any related ethical, rehabilitation, neurobiological or specialized diagnostic issues which arise. Although neurology is practised predominantly in outpatients nowadays, students should take every opportunity to study those patients who are admitted to hospital with disabling or acute neurological disease. Such patients offer the opportunity to take histories of classic and important conditions, such as subarachnoid haemorrhage, cerebral infarction, meningitis or spinal cord compression. Furthermore, it is such patients who are most likely to display abnormal physical signs. A single observation of papilloedema, nystagmus, ataxia or an extensor plantar response indelibly imprints itself on the student's mind.

Neurology encompasses all the interesting aspects of modern medicine. Clinical skills remain fundamental to diagnosis and are backed up by sophisticated and precise investigations such as magnetic resonance imaging. Contrary to the popular belief that neurological disease is generally untreatable, a wide range of therapies are used nowadays in everyday practice, to treat such varied conditions as epilepsy, movement disorders, headaches, neuromuscular disease, infections, and cerebrovascular disease. Exciting new therapies are being developed for multiple sclerosis and neurodegenerative disorders. Ethical issues arise in everyday practice, ranging from decisions about how much and when to tell patients of incurable disease, to confronting the genetic implications of certain diagnoses. Increasingly refined rehabilitation techniques are available for physically or psychologically disabled patients. Molecular science is proving immensely powerful in unravelling the pathogenesis of neurological diseases, and in opening novel therapeutic avenues.

Students transferring from preclinical study of the nervous system often feel that the excitement of modern neurobiology has little application to the everyday neurological problems they encounter during their clinical studies. It is an inescapable fact that a good working knowledge of gross neuroanatomy, and its relation to functional localization, provides the basis for many clinical neurological diagnoses. Accordingly, this book revises some crucial neuroanatomical and neurophysiological knowledge required by students. But we are beginning to understand neurological diseases in terms of disordered cell biology. So far, this approach has generally been applied to diseases which are rare, and often genetic. Some such disorders are discussed in this book so as to introduce the new manner in which we will think about the pathogenesis of many neurological diseases in the future.

I am deeply indebted to many for their help, both direct and indirect, in preparing this book. Anne Richardson prepared the manuscript with her inimitable combination of skill, speed, and humour. Daren Forward and Nick White were unstinting and forgiving partners in preparing the illustrations. Valuable material for figures was generously provided by P. Anslow, J. Byrne, J. Elston, M. Esiri, B. Gardiner, R. Kennett, K. Mills, A. Molyneux, G. Quaghebeur, and S. Wallace. Inspiration is currently undervalued as an educational force; my own enthusiasm for neurology, and for the clinical method, was inspired by K. Citron, C.J. Earl, J. Gawler, the late R.W. Gilliatt, M.J.G. Harrison, J.G.G. Ledingham, J. Marshall, P.K. Thomas and J.Z. Young. Finally, I would like to thank the staff of the Oxford University Press for encouraging me to write this book, and for their skilful production work.

Oxford, March 1997   Michael Donaghy

Contents

CHAPTER 1

History taking

Chapter contents

Common neurological conditions

Almost 10 per cent of the population consult their general practitioner about a neurological symptom each year in the UK, and less than 10 per cent of these are referred for a specialist opinion. The commonest conditions seen by neurologists are shown in Table 1.1. Together they account for roughly 75 per cent of neurological symptomology. Usually they are diagnosed on clinical grounds. All doctors should be aware of the clinical approach to these problems.

The other 25 per cent of neurological disorders include a huge diversity of diseases, many rare. These include many serious conditions such as brain tumours, infections, and neurodegenerative diseases. These rarer disorders are particularly likely to require highly specialized advice about investigation, treatment, prognosis, and genetic implications. Some

TABLE 1.1 The commonest conditions seen by neurologists
Headache and face pain
Blackouts and epilepsy
Peripheral nerve and root disorders
Cerebrovascular disease
Multiple sclerosis
Parkinsonism and movement disorders
Dementia
Giddiness and vertigo
Psychologically determined symptoms

of these conditions, although rare, are eminently treatable, such as myasthenia gravis.

History taking

History taking is the cornerstone of neurological diagnosis. It tends to be more informative than examination, which usually merely confirms information anticipated by the history. But sometimes examination is particularly helpful. For instance, in localizing the anatomical abnormality responsible for muscle weakness, specific physical signs reveal whether it is the upper motor neuron, the lower motor neuron, or the muscle which is diseased. Unexpected discovery of physical signs such as extensor plantar responses, signifying pyramidal tract damage, or papilloedema, signifying raised intracranial pressure, crucially alter one's view if the history has suggested diagnoses such as psychologically determined weakness or benign tension headache.

A good history provides a story whose internal direction points intuitively towards a diagnosis. It is much more revealing to treat the history as story telling than to take the utilitarian approach of simply listing symptoms and expect a diagnosis to appear miraculously. Experience allows one to recognize that patients often describe the symptoms of certain disorders in a very characteristic manner. There is no particular list of questions to ask. You should invite the patient to describe their symptoms in the order in which they occurred. Important details are clarified by asking specific questions during or after the patient's account. It is useful to determine whether a patient's symptoms are sufficiently 'disabling' to prevent crucial everyday activities or work, or whether they are merely a 'nuisance'. This will help you to decide whether a symptom such as headache needs treatment.

Background history

Conventional teaching is to enquire about the background history after recording the presenting complaint. But it is often more helpful to the overall consultation to start with the background medical, family, drug, and social histories before moving on to the patient's presenting complaint. This is easily introduced by saying 'Your doctor has asked if I would see you because of x (e.g. dizziness), but I wonder if I could ask you a few background questions about your health first.' This can produce a myriad of information relevant to how you interpret and pursue the subsequent symptoms of the presenting complaint. For instance, the discovery that a patient with limb tinglings has diabetes makes diabetic neuropathy likely, or that a patient with a seizure may be taking a tricyclic antidepressant drug which is known to lower seizure thresholds, or

someone with a choreiform movement disorder may have had a demented parent thereby raising the question of dominantly inherited Huntington's chorea.

But there are two other powerful reasons for early enquiry about the patient's background. First, by showing your interest in a patient, for instance, by discussing their employment or family, you can establish the foundation for empathy. This helps a patient make the crucial decision about whether to trust you to advise them about their medical condition. Secondly, you can find out about the way in which a patient reacts to their own background and to your simple questions. For instance, are their answers straightforward, meandering, lacking in insight, or downright devious? Are they pessimistic or optimistic, philosophical or blameful, open or suspicious? And by observing the manner whereby patients answer enquiries about everyday matters, and comparing this with how they subsequently react to questions about their illness, it becomes easier to detect the inconsistent or discordant answers of someone who is manufacturing their symptoms psychologically, a common diagnosis in neurology.

Some aspects of the neurological history provide important pointers to the diagnosis. However, your enquiry about them should be couched in terms that do not prejudice the patient's answer. Table 1.2 summarizes the general principles of history taking.

Time course

Sudden or instantaneous onset of symptoms usually indicates epilepsy (abrupt loss of consciousness) or cerebrovascular disease (the instantaneous headache of subarachnoid haemorrhage, or the sudden hemiparesis due to middle cerebral artery embolus). Symptoms that deter-

TABLE 1.2	General principles of history taking

1 Enquire about the patient's background (employment, family, habits, medication, past medical history, family history, general health).

2 Ask the patient to describe their symptoms in the order in which they occurred.

3 Then, if necessary, enquire about:

> Time course
> Negative or positive symptoms
> Anatomical localizations
> Eye witness account
> Previous neurological history
> Family history

iorate subacutely, over hours, days, or even a few weeks, are generally caused by inflammatory or demyelinating disorders. **Steadily** worsening symptoms over months or years may indicate the growth of a tumour, or a neuro-degenerative process. **Relapsing and remitting** symptoms, which come and go over a few weeks, are typical of multiple sclerosis, whilst recurring headaches, each lasting 3 hours to 3 days, are typical of migraine.

Negative and positive symptoms

Negative symptoms are those in which normal neuro-logical functions are lost. This is the commonest type of symptom caused by damage to the nervous system. Examples include the hemiparesis due to cerebral hemisphere infarction, the memory loss due to Alzheimer's disease, muscle weakness due to motor neuron degeneration, or the loss of sphincter control due to cauda equina tumour.

Positive symptoms are novel phenomena which often suggest specific diagnoses. Flashing lights (photopsia) or zig-zag lines (fortification spectra) preceding a headache are diagnostic of migraine. A hallucination of a peculiar smell, often resembling burning rubber, is the typical uncinate hallucination of an epileptic discharge in the temporal lobe. Repetitive twitching of the fingers occurs in focal motor seizures. Tingling in the fingers and toes is typical of acquired rather than inherited disorders of peripheral nerve sensory fibres. A 'pill-rolling' tremor of the fingers at rest is diagnostic of Parkinsonism.

Anatomical localization

Sometimes you must enquire about other symptoms in order to localize the disease process anatomically. For instance, ask the patient with suspected motor neuron disease to confirm that there are no sensory or sphincter symptoms that might point to generalized peripheral nerve disease or to compression of the spinal cord. Ask a patient with sensory symptoms in the legs whether their hands are also affected; this would be a pointer to a polyneuropathy rather than a focal lesion of the cauda equina or thoracic spinal cord. Determine whether a patient with dysphasia also has loss of spatial abilities, such as a dressing apraxia or getting lost in familiar places; this would point to a generalized dementing process involving both cerebral hemispheres rather than a focal lesion of the left hemisphere causing pure dysphasia. Enquire whether a patient with gait unsteadiness also has vertigo or double vision, which imply a lesion of the brainstem rather than of the cerebellum or the sensory pathways in the spinal cord or peripheral nerves.

Eye witness accounts

Patients with generalized epilepsy cannot recall what they did whilst unconscious and often cannot recollect the onset of the blackout. So an eye witness account of a generalized convulsion or automatic behaviour is generally more use than electroencephalography in diagnosing epilepsy. In a patient with poor memory and insight due to early dementia, it is often the spouse who provides the evidence for loss of intellectual function: forgetting grandchildren's names, personality change, or loss of ability to do the usual crossword. Patients with motor neuron disease are often unaware of the fasciculations in their limb muscles, yet their spouse may have felt them occurring whilst in bed.

Previous neurological history

This is crucial for establishing the diagnosis of multiple sclerosis, which is a disorder of the central nervous system which is disseminated in space and time. Thus, eliciting a history of unilateral visual loss due to optic neuritis a decade earlier suggests multiple sclerosis in a middle-aged patient with gait unsteadiness and sensory disturbance on the arm and trunk due to a spinal cord lesion.

Family history

There are many inherited neurological disorders, although individually they are usually rare. In patients with long-standing wasting and weakness below the knees, and with high foot arches (pes cavus), enquiry revealing autosomal dominant inheritance of a similar disorder in the family is diagnostic of hereditary motor and sensory neuropathy, otherwise known as Charcot–Marie–Tooth disease. First-cousin marriage between the parents may be a clue to autosomal recessive disorders in offspring with neurological disorders. Sex-linked recessive disorders, which are transmitted via the X chromosome and occur only in males, do not manifest in the mother, but may be present in the males of earlier or parallel generations.

Coexisting medical disorders

Progressively deteriorating neurological symptoms should provoke enquiry about possible underlying cancer which might be involving the nervous system: smoking history, weight loss, chest symptoms, bowel symptoms, and recent breast and gynaecological check-ups. In a patient with **cerebrovascular disease**, a history of valvular or ischaemic heart disease, hypertension, diabetes, oral contraceptive usage, or even cocaine abuse may be important. Unusual neurological diseases, such as opportunistic infections or central nervous system lymphoma, must be considered in the increasing numbers of **immunocompromised** patients who have received organ transplants, or are HIV infected. Typical **medication side-effects** include headache, vertigo, tremor, tinglings, and peripheral neuropathy. A patient's drugs should be checked in a formulary for such side-effects, and the timing of the symptoms compared with that of the drug's usage. The **travel history** may raise the possibility that a patient's neurological symptoms are due to infections such as schistosomiasis, malaria, diphtheria, or borreliosis. Patients **addicted** to alcohol or recreational drugs are notorious for underestimating or denying consumption; this may be directly relevant to explaining ataxia, memory loss, peripheral neuropathy, or muscle weakness in the case of alcohol, and stroke or seizures in the case of cocaine.

CASE 1.1 'A RISKY APPROACH TO THE DOCTOR–PATIENT RELATIONSHIP'

A young married woman was admitted because of subarachnoid haemorrhage. The onset of pain had been instantaneous 'as though I had been kicked in the head'. Fortunately she remained fully conscious and lucid, with only minor neck stiffness and photophobia. A potential candidate for early clipping of her cerebral aneurism, we arranged a consultation with the neurosurgeon. The diagnosis was not in doubt, and as an opening gambit he asked when the headache had come on. 'Around 11 o'clock on Sunday morning' came the reply. 'And what were you doing?' he asked. 'I was in bed, you know . . . , with my husband', she replied in somewhat meaningful tones. The surgeon, also a man of conviction, glanced at the gold crucifix on her necklace and with a friendly smile he commented wryly, 'Perhaps if you'd gone to church this wouldn't have happened.' There was a short hesitation during which the hearts were in the mouths of the accompanying doctors and nurses. Fortunately she saw the humorous side to his somewhat risky, indeed risqué, comment and she laughed. Next day he clipped her aneurism with his usual skill, and she returned happily to her usual vigorous life.

Comment

- Some diseases are described in such characteristic terms that you should record them verbatim in your history. Typical examples are the description of subarachnoid haemorrhage as '*being kicked in the head*', of tension headache as '*like a tight hat*', or of a classical migraine aura as '*coloured zig-zag lines*'.

- There is no doubt that humour, if used correctly, can be a valuable vehicle in enabling a patient and doctor to lay down the foundations of personal understanding and trust which underpin a successful doctor–patient relationship. In particular, patients appreciate the relationship being put on an easy footing which gives them the ability to talk freely about their concerns.

- But the brand of humour is all-important. If it is sympathetic or kindly ironic, it is unlikely to cause offence. However, an attempt at being funny can be disastrous if it appears to be a glib substitute for taking the patient seriously, if it is scathing or sneering, if it implies blame, or if it plays to the gallery of medical and nursing colleagues at the expense of the patient. It was clear from the manner of the moment that our neurosurgeon was being kindly ironic, rather than playing to the gallery.

- The manner in which you take the history can be particularly liable to misinterpretation in circumstances such as these, where the illness had clearly been precipitated by a private activity of exquisite personal value to the patient. In particular one must avoid making a patient feel guilty about the cause of their illness, and try to prevent them harbouring inhibitions about the safety of resuming a blamed activity even after successful treatment to remove the risk of recurrence.

CHAPTER 2

A basic neurological examination

Chapter contents

Many students and doctors never acquire competence in neurological examination because they are put off by the enormously long list of manoeuvres that could be performed. However, it is easy to learn a basic neurological examination which takes only a few minutes. The following description of such an examination addresses practical issues such as which instructions to give, where to put your hands for best effect, and how to interpret fundamentals such as abnormal reflexes. This basic examination is perfectly sufficient for examining the patient with uncomplicated headache or epilepsy, or as part of a general medical examination for the patient without neurological symptoms. This basic examination concentrates on manoeuvres that give unequivocal evidence of pathology, such as looking for papilloedema, tone changes, or extensor plantar responses. It avoids manoeuvres that are simply repetitive or imprecise ways of detecting the same pathology.

Other tests should be added to this examination if the patient's symptoms suggest a particular disorder, if abnormalities requiring further evaluation crop up during the basic examination, or if one is asked to examine a specific feature under exam conditions, such as vision or a weak limb.

The basic examination should be performed in four stages: first during history taking, second whilst the patient is walking, third whilst sitting, and fourth whilst the patient is lying down (Table 2.1).

TABLE 2.1   A basic neurological examination
During history taking, examine
Speech and cognition
Facial expression
Involuntary movements
Stand the patient up and examine
Gait
Heel–toe walking
Romberg test
With the patient sitting facing you, examine
Cranial nerves
◆ Fundoscopy
◆ Visual fields
◆ Horizontal eye movements
◆ Pupil–light responses
◆ Facial sensation
◆ Facial movements
◆ Hearing
◆ Palatal movement
◆ Tongue movement
The arms
◆ Inspection
◆ Tone
◆ Power (shoulder abduction and finger spreading)
◆ Finger–nose coordination
Lie patient down and examine
Arm reflexes (biceps and triceps)
The legs
◆ Inspection
◆ Ankle clonus
◆ Power (hip flexion and ankle dorsiflexion)
◆ Reflexes (knee and ankle)
◆ Plantar responses
Finally, examine additional features suggested by the history or by abnormalities on the basic examination

Examination during history taking

Whilst taking the history observe three things:

1 **Speech and cognition**. Abnormalities of speech, thought, or memory raise the question of dysphasia or generalized dementia. Dysarthic speech is slurred. Dysphonic speech is quiet.

2 **The range of facial expression**. An impassive face suggests Parkinson's disease, or occasionally bilateral facial palsy. A sad face suggests depression. Dementia diminishes non-verbal communication by facial expression and gesture.

3 **Involuntary movements**. Pill-rolling tremor of the fingers at rest is typical of Parkinson's disease. Sudden choreiform movements of the hands occur in Huntington's disease, and may look like fidgets or be disguised as mannerisms. Spasms of unilateral eye closure occur in hemifacial spasm. Fixed or spasmodic head rotation occurs in torticollis.

Examination with the patient standing

Gait

In the wide-based gait of ataxia the feet cross more than the usual 5 cm apart, and the stride length is irregular. Uniformly small strides occur in the gait apraxia of frontal-lobe disease. Difficulty in starting, shuffling,

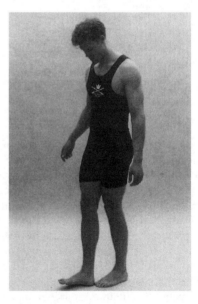

Fig. 2.1 Heel–toe walking.

and then progressively lengthening strides occur in Parkinsonism. Arm swing is lost in Parkinson's disease, usually unilaterally early on. Floppy foot drops occur in peripheral nerve or nerve root disease. Stiff foot drops occur in spastic upper motor neuron lesions, or occasionally in dystonia. A waddling gait, with drop of the pelvis on the striding side, occurs in proximal muscle weakness due to myopathy.

Heel–toe walking

This is an excellent screening test for cerebellar disease, or sensorimotor abnormalities affecting the limbs. It is best tested by saying 'I would like you to walk heel-to-toe, like this' and demonstrating two or three such steps (Fig. 2.1). Patients will be unable to do this without stumbling to the side if they have ataxia due to cerebellar disease, or loss of proprioception due to peripheral neuropathy or dorsal column disease.

The Romberg test

This is a quick and excellent screen for loss of proprioceptive feedback from the legs in peripheral neuropathy or spinal cord disease (Fig. 2.2). In patients with abnormal heel–toe walking, it will distinguish those patients with ataxia due to loss of proprioceptive feedback from those with ataxia due to cerebellar disease. It is best tested by saying 'stand with your feet together, get your bearings, and now close your eyes—I won't let you fall', whilst preparing to steady the patient's shoulders with your hands if he starts toppling.

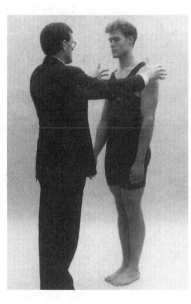

Fig. 2.2 Romberg test.

This test is positive if the patient falls, or is unable to maintain balance without corrective movements of the feet. It is important to realize that a proper Romberg test is not merely testing balance with the eyes closed, but compares stability with and without visual feedback.

A truly positive Romberg test takes some moments to develop, with an increasing amplitude of slow swaying until a critical degree of lean occurs, beyond which the patient can no longer remain upright. Not uncommonly one encounters patients who promptly fall in one direction immediately upon closing their eyes; this usually results from lack of confidence or is other-wise psychologically determined, and rarely indicates structural disease of the nervous system.

Examination with the patient sitting

Cranial nerves

Ophthalmoscopy

Inspect the optic nerve head, also called the optic disc. Everybody finds this difficult at first, principally because they 'get lost within the eye' and can't find the optic disc. It helps to use a familiar ophthalmoscope, and one whose optics haven't been misaligned by being dropped. But the most important thing is to understand the position of the optic nerve head (which corresponds to the blind spot) within the visual field and its corresponding position in the eye. Then you can set up the correct geometry so that you can look into the eye confident that you will be looking directly at, or very near to, the optic disc. The following method is infallible and should be practised on a colleague until it becomes second nature.

1 You should know that the blind spot, which represents the optic disc, lies about 20° of visual angle lateral to the point of fixation in each eye (Fig. 2.3, on next page). Also it lies just below the horizontal. This determines your 'line of attack'.

2 Ask the patient to fixate on a point behind you which is chosen for height so that you are comfortably able to look into their eye from just below its horizontal meridian. The particular fixation point you choose for the patient will depend upon the relative heights of your own and the patient's head.

3 Using the ophthalmoscope on your right eye to examine the patient's right eye, and vice versa for the left, look into the eye from about 20° lateral

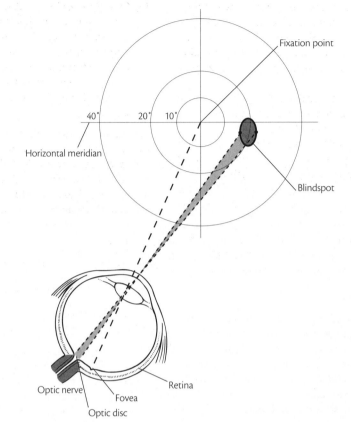

Fig. 2.3 The blind spot of the right eye, its position in the visual field, and its relationship to the optic disc inside the eyeball.

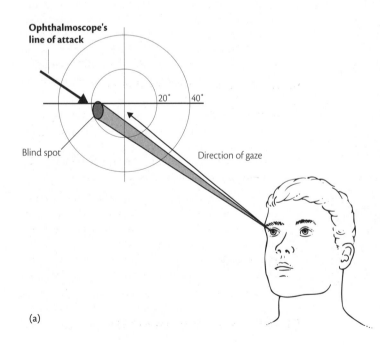

(a)

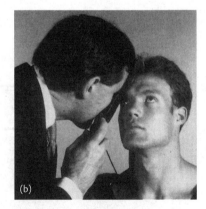

(b)

Fig. 2.4 The 'line of attack' for ophthalmoscopy when looking at the right optic disc. (a) Diagrammatic representation. (b) Note that the patient's other eye is maintaining the direction of fixation.

to the line of fixation, and from just below the horizontal (Fig. 2.4). Examine whether the edge of the optic disc is **sharply defined** as is normal, or has **blurred edges** suggesting disc swelling due to papilloedema due to raised intracranial pressure.

(a) The **normal optic disc** (Fig. 2.5) is yellow–pink in colour, has sharply defined edges, and the blood vessels run flatly across the edge.

(b) In **moderate papilloedema** (Fig. 2.6), the edges of the optic disc are swollen, bending the blood vessels forwards. Sometimes the calibre of the blood vessels narrows as they pass through the oedematous disc edge, and the veins become engorged.

(c) In **severe papilloedema** (Fig. 2.7), haemorrhages and cotton wool spots appear around the edge of the optic disc in addition to the changes of moderate papilloedema.

(d) In **optic atrophy** (Fig. 2.8), the optic disc becomes white. In primary optic atrophy the edges of the disc are sharp and the underlying cause is usually optic neuritis, occlusion of the central retinal artery, or trauma or compression of the optic nerve. In optic atrophy secondary to chronic papilloedema, the edges of the optic disc are blurred.

4 Having inspected the optic disc, you can inspect the vessels and more peripheral parts of the retina, for instance, if diabetic retinopathy is suspected (Fig. 2.9). If you wish to look at the foveal pit, or macula, you should ask the patient to stare directly at the spot of a narrow ophthalmoscope beam.

Visual fields

Detailed examination of the peripheral and central portions of the visual fields of each eye separately is time-consuming and rarely rewarding unless the

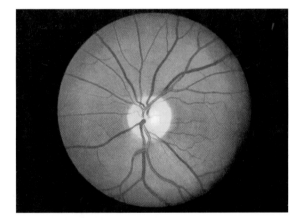

Fig. 2.5 The normal optic disc.

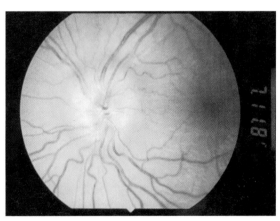

Fig. 2.6 The optic disc in moderate papilloedema.

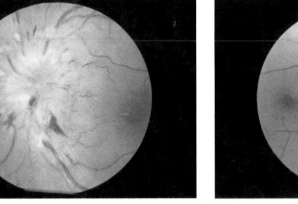

Fig. 2.7 The optic disc in severe papilloedema.

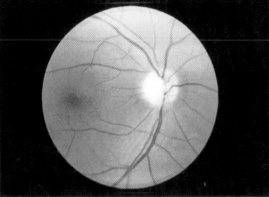

Fig. 2.8 The optic disc in primary optic atrophy.

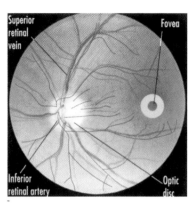

Fig. 2.9 Diagram of retinal structures seen at fundoscopy.

patient has visual symptoms or pituitary disease. As a simple screen for **homonymous hemianopia** (which is an identical visual field deficit in both eyes due to cerebral hemisphere disease) (Fig. 14.2 p. 99), and for **sensory inattention** (due to parietal lobe lesions) the following quick manoeuvre is recommended. Ask the patient to 'keep your eyes fixed on my nose and point to whichever of my index fingers moves'. Then raise your arms so as to place your index fingers at about 80° peripheral in each visual field. After keeping still for a moment flick the tip of one index finger once whilst keeping the rest of your arm still. The patient should immediately point to the side that moved (Fig. 2.10).

Sensory inattention may be detected by moving your finger on both sides simultaneously, but the patient will only see movement on one side. Of course sensory inattention, which reflects a parietal lobe lesion, can only be diagnosed if each visual field is normal when tested separately.

Eye movements

First, look at the patient's face when he is looking straight ahead to see if there is a droopy eyelid, known as ptosis. This is easier to detect when unilateral. In a definite ptosis, the eyelid will overlap the edge of the pupil when the patient is looking straight ahead.

Ask the patient 'to hold your chin with one hand [so as to prevent head movements] and then follow my finger with your eyes'. Hold a stick or your finger vertically and move it laterally to about 50° or 60°. Hold it still for a moment whilst asking the patient whether he sees it as single or double. Simultaneously inspect the eyes closely to detect the jerking movements called nystagmus or for any paralysis of ocular movement (Fig. 2.11). Then repeat this procedure to the other side.

Then test vertical eye movements by holding your finger horizontally and moving it up and then down by about 45°, once again enquiring for diplopia and observing for nystagmus (Fig. 2.12). You may need to hold the eyelids up so as to see the eye position in downgaze.

Pupils

To test the pupil–light reflex, first ask the patient to fixate your nose and note the size of the pupils before light stimulation (Fig. 2.13(a)). If it is very difficult to see the pupil because of dim illumination, or a darkly pig-

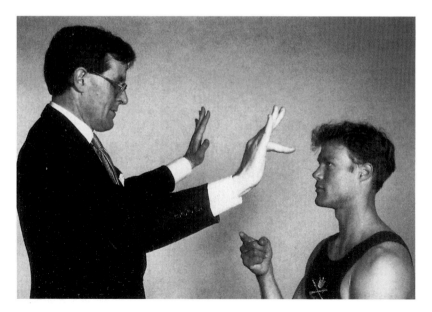

Fig. 2.10 Visual field testing by simple confrontation. The patient's eyes fixate the examiner's nose. The examiner's hands should be placed stationary, about 80° peripheral in each visual field.

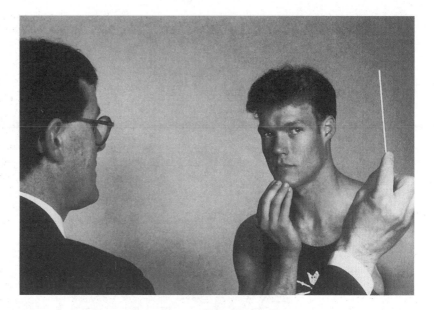

Fig. 2.11 Testing horizontal eye movements: observe for nystagmus or an ocular palsy and ask whether there is double vision.

mented iris, it helps to shine the torch beam at the bridge of the nose (Fig. 2.13(a) so that light scatter makes the pupil visible, without stimulating the pupil–light response.

Second, shine a torch directly into the left eye and observe that both pupils constrict equally (Fig. 2.13(b)). This elicits the direct pupil–light response on the left and the indirect (or consensual) response on the right.

Third, swing the torch beam quickly across to the right eye and check that there is no further dilatation or con-striction of either pupil (Fig. 2.13(c)). This allows compari-son of the direct and consensual pupil responses of each eye. If there were an optic nerve lesion on the right, both pupils would dilate slightly when the torch was shone into the right eye, compared with their normal constric-tion following left eye stimulation. This way of testing the pupils has the sensitivity to detect relative, rather than absolute, afferent pupillary defects due to partial optic nerve lesions, for instance, resulting from optic neuritis. The pupil–light reflex is an example of a 'unilat-eral afferent–bilateral efferent' reflex (p. 12).

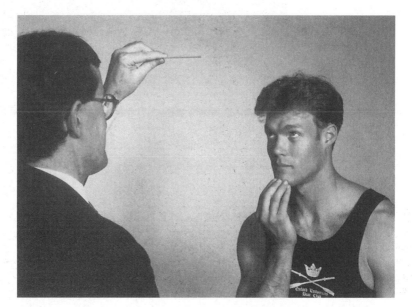

Fig. 2.12 Testing upgaze.

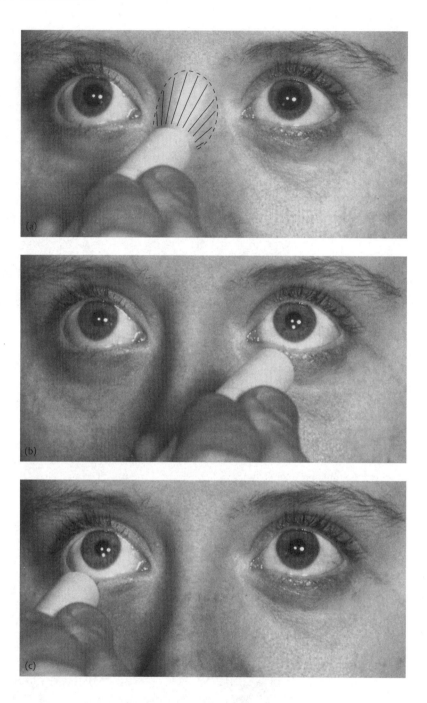

Fig. 2.13 Testing the pupil–light reflex using the 'swinging torch' method.

The commonest cause of a unilaterally small pupil is damage to the cervical sympathetic pathway (Horner's syndrome) (Fig. 2.14), which will be associated with a slight degree of eyelid drooping (ptosis).

A unilaterally fixed and dilated pupil is typical of an oculomotor nerve lesion (cranial III), in which there will also be impairment of adduction and vertical eye movement, and a more marked ptosis (Fig. 2.15).

Facial sensation

Run the finger tips of both your hands simultaneously across the patient's forehead, onto the cheek and nose,

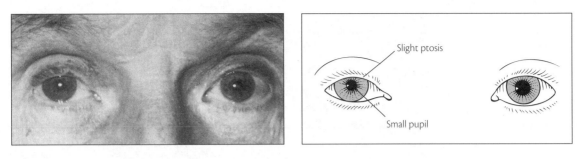

Fig. 2.14 Horner's syndrome.

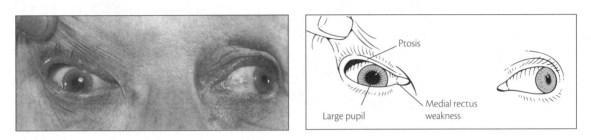

Fig. 2.15 Third nerve palsy.

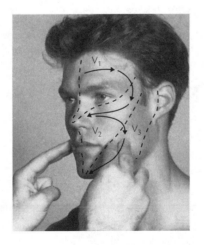

Fig. 2.16 Testing facial sensation.

and then onto the chin (Fig. 2.16). Whilst doing so, ask 'do my fingers feel like fingers and the same on each side?' as you cover all three territories of the trigeminal nerve, frontal (V_1), maxillary (V_2), and mandibular (V_3). Any area of altered sensation can be tested and mapped out using a pin or cotton wool wisp.

Testing the **corneal reflex** is not necessary as a routine. The following method is recommended if you do need to test the corneal reflex, for instance, if you suspect potentially harmful loss of corneal sensation or a subtle facial nerve lesion. Make a fine wisp of cotton wool and ask the patient to look upwards whilst

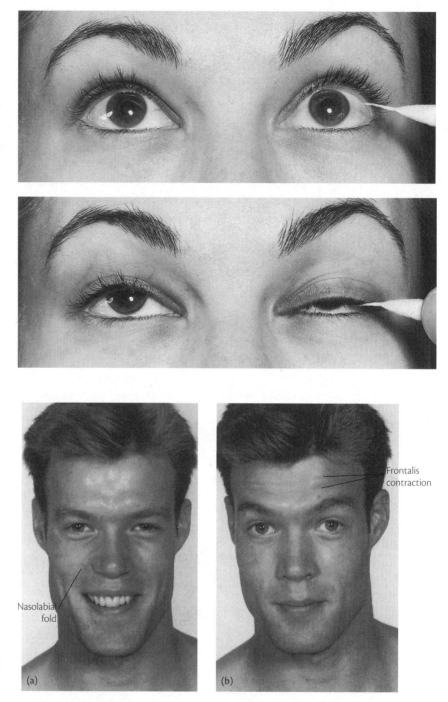

Fig. 2.17 Testing the corneal reflex by touching the edge of the cornea with a wisp of cotton wool on one side (top), and observing blinking of both eyes (bottom).

Fig. 2.18 Testing facial movements: (a) mouth 'give me a smile'; (b) forehead 'raise your eyebrows'.

warning them that 'I'm going to touch the corner of your eye with this cotton wool.' Introduce this cotton wisp from below and to the side and brush the junction between the cornea and sclera (Fig. 2.17). Normally a unilateral stimulus provokes bilateral blinking, another example of a 'unilateral afferent–bilateral efferent' reflex (p. 27). Contact lenses are the commonest cause of seemingly absent corneal reflexes.

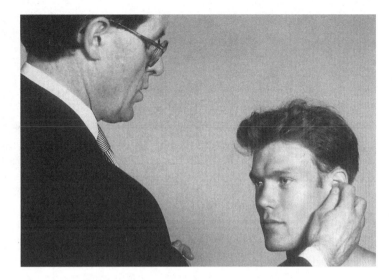

Fig. 2.19 Testing hearing in the right ear with a whisper. The left ear is masked by rubbing a finger in the external auditory meatus.

Facial movements

Step back two or three paces so that you can see both sides of the patient's mouth simultaneously. Then say 'show me your teeth like this' or 'give me a smile'. It helps to smile at the patient while you give the instruction; often they respond with an involuntary grin which demonstrates facial movements perfectly. Observe whether both sides of the mouth move equally quickly, and produce similar elevation and deepening of the nasolabial skin creases (2.18(a)).

If the movement is asymmetrical, hold back the patient's fringe and ask him to 'raise your eyebrows' to see whether both sides of the frontalis muscle in the forehead contract equally (Fig. 2.18(b)).

Lower motor neuron lesions of the seventh nerve affect movement of both forehead and mouth. Unilateral upper motor neuron facial paralysis affects only the mouth and lower face, but not the forehead.

Hearing

Say to the patient 'Could you repeat this number' whilst whispering a number from a distance of about 2 feet (60 cm) to test hearing in their right ear whilst lightly rubbing the tip of your finger in the left ear to create a masking noise (Fig. 2.19).

Then reverse the masking and test the left ear. Unilateral or bilateral deafness should be examined further by Weber's and Rinne's tests to determine whether it is conductive or sensorineural deafness (see Chapter 15), and by auroscopic examination of the eardrum.

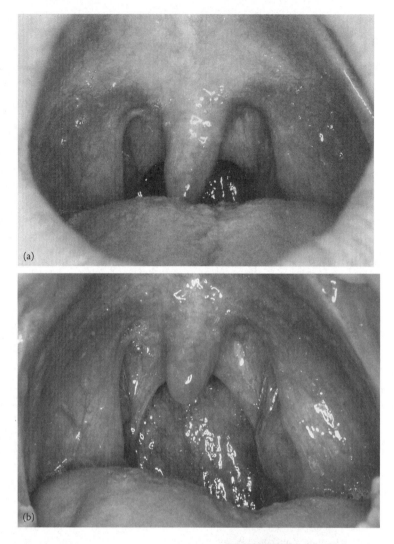

Fig. 2.20 (a) The palate at rest; (b) elevation of the palate and uvula on saying 'ah'.

Palatal movements

Ask the patient to open their mouth and say 'ah' whilst illuminating the throat with a torch (Fig. 2.20). There is no need to elicit the gag reflex routinely if the elevation of the palate and uvula is normal and symmetrical, and there is no swallowing difficulty or dysphonia. The gag reflex is uncomfortable, but is elicited when necessary by stimulating each side of the soft palate with an orange stick and watching the resultant rise of both sides of the palate. The gag reflex is also an example of a 'unilateral afferent–bilateral efferent' reflex (p. 27).

Tongue movement

Observe the tongue for wasting or fasciculations while it is resting on the floor of the mouth during examination of palatal movements. Don't look for fasciculations

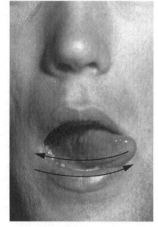

Fig. 2.21 Alternating tongue movements.

whilst the tongue is being actively protruded since most normal tongues show ripples and flickers under such circumstances. Then ask the patient to 'stick out your tongue and waggle it from side to side like this' (as you yourself demonstrate) (Fig. 2.21).

Lower motor neuron lesions of a hypoglossal nerve lead to the tongue wasting on, and deviating towards, the same side as the lesion (Fig. 2.22). In bilateral upper motor neuron lesions, the tongue becomes spastic and pointed and its movement is slow and limited. In a cerebellar lesion, alternating tongue movements will be slowed and irregular, in other words ataxic.

The arms

Inspection

The patient should sit facing you on the edge of the couch whilst you observe the contour of the shoulders and upper arms for **muscle wasting** or fasciculations. The hands should be inspected for muscle wasting. Look particularly at the first dorsal interosseous muscles on the dorsum of the hand between the thumb and forefinger, which are innervated by the ulnar nerve, and at the abductor policis brevis in the lateral part of the thenar eminence, which is innervated by the median nerve.

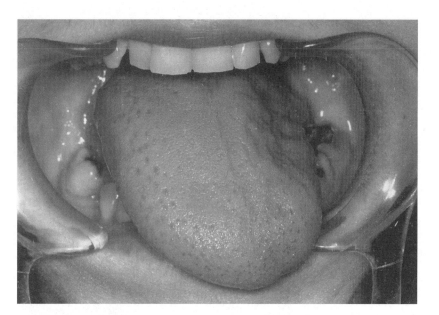

Fig. 2.22 Left tongue hemiatrophy due to a hypoglossal nerve lesion.

Tone

Both the extrapyramidal rigidity of Parkinson's disease, and the spasticity associated with an upper motor neuron lesion can be detected reliably in the arms. The exact method you use to test tone is determined by which of these conditions is suspected.

Spasticity should be sought by holding the patient's hand, and abruptly supinating the forearm to detect a sudden jerk of resistance called a '**pronator catch**' (Fig. 2.23).

The '**cog-wheel rigidity**' of Parkinson's disease is best sought by holding the patient's wrist with one hand, and repeatedly flexing and extending the fingers and wrist by gripping the tips of the fingers with your other hand (Fig. 2.24). The term 'cog-wheel rigidity' merely describes the combination of leadpipe rigidity and a superimposed tremor.

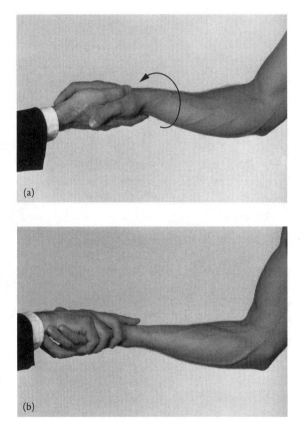

Fig. 2.23 Testing for a pronator catch in the right arm: (a) starting position (pronation); (b) finishing position (supination).

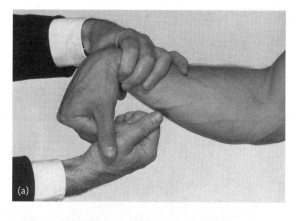

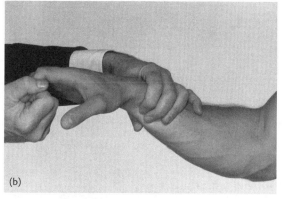

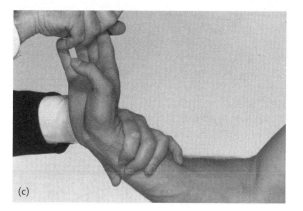

Fig. 2.24 Testing for cog-wheel rigidity in Parkinson's disease.

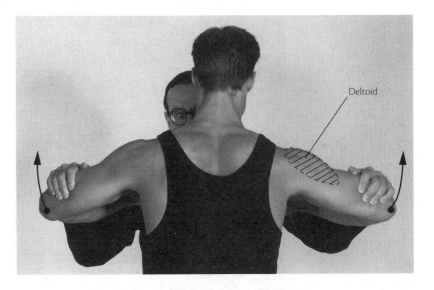

Fig. 2.25 Testing shoulder abduction power (deltoid).

Power

For general screening purposes it is sufficient to test one proximal and one distal muscle in each arm. Additional muscles are tested if clinically indicated: for instance, if you suspect a lesion of a particular peripheral nerve or root.

A good proximal muscle to test is **shoulder abduction** to 90° by deltoid (C5 root, axillary nerve) (Fig. 2.25).

A good distal muscle to test is the **first dorsal interosseous** (TI root, ulnar nerve), which spreads the fingers apart (Fig. 2.26). Its power can be compared with one's own first dorsal interosseous.

Coordination

The finger–nose test is only sensitive if the patient is required to stretch their arm out fully so as to reach the examiner's target finger. The examiner should stand immediately behind his own target finger for the best detection of any randomly distributed inaccuracies in the patient's pointing known as ataxia or dysmetria (Fig. 2.27).

Dysmetria on the finger–nose test usually indicates cerebellar disease (**cerebellar ataxia**), or loss of proprioceptive feedback (**sensory ataxia**). The sensory form of ataxia is usually associated with pseudoathetosis in which the outstretched fingers wander when the eyes are closed (Fig. 2.28).

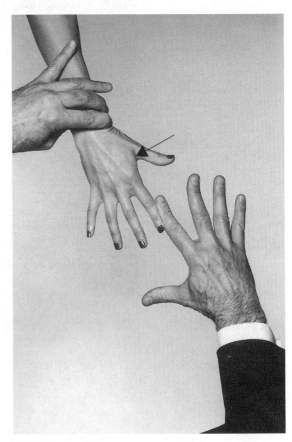

Fig. 2.26 Testing finger abduction power (dorsal interrosseous). The examiner compares the power of his abducted index finger with that of the patient. The bulk of the patient's first interosseous muscle is clearly visible (arrow).

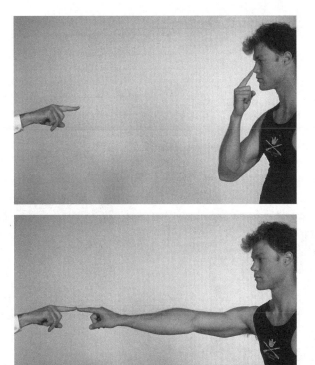

Fig. 2.27 The finger–nose test to detect dysmetria (ataxia).

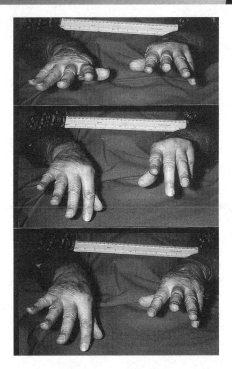

Fig. 2.28 Pseudoathetosis in a patient with sensory ataxic polyneuropathy. Frame intervals at 30 sec.

Examination with the patient lying down

Arm tendon reflexes

Now the patient should lie down, and the **biceps reflex** (musculocutaneous nerve; C5, C6 roots) should be tested from the right side. Put your thumb on the tendon to transmit a firm blow from the tendon hammer to the biceps tendon within the cramped space of the antecubital fossa to elicit a visible and palpable contraction of the biceps muscle (Fig. 2.29).

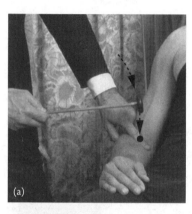

(a)

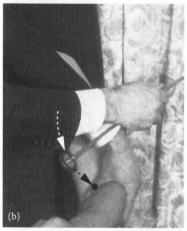

(b)

Fig. 2.29 Eliciting (a) the right and then (b) the left biceps tendon reflexes (C5/C6).

Then test the **triceps reflex** (radial nerve; C7, C8 roots). Because the triceps muscle has an extremely short tendon, the hammerhead should hit the tendon at right angles just above the elbow (Fig. 2.30).

Testing the brachioradialis reflex (radial nerve; C6 root) rarely adds extra information to that obtained from the biceps reflex unless an isolated lesion of the C6 root or radical nerve root is suspected.

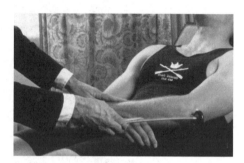

Fig. 2.30 Eliciting the triceps reflex (C7/C8).

Interpreting tendon reflexes

Tendon reflexes are **brisk** in upper motor neuron lesions. An **absent** tendon reflex will be due to a peripheral nerve or nerve root lesion. Before finally declaring a reflex to be absent you should carry out **reinforcement**. This is most easily achieved by asking the patient to 'bite your teeth together when I say "bite"', whilst you simultaneously swing the tendon hammer to try and elicit the reflex.

The legs

Observation

You should stand at the end of the couch so as to view each leg equally for wasting. Ask the patient to 'tighten your kneecaps'. This allows the bulk of the vastus medialis component of quadriceps to be assessed just above and medial to the knee (Fig. 2.31). Then examine distal muscles by asking the patient to 'cock your toes towards you' and check that the tibialis anterior muscle bulges proud of the anterior border of the tibial bone.

The leg muscles should be observed for **fasciculations** and the skin for **trophic changes**. Fasciculations are visible as flickering contractions within the muscle belly, which are insufficient to produce movement at the joint. They signify disease of the lower motor neuron, such as motor neuron disease. Trophic changes consist of skin ulcers, burns, or disrupted joints (Charcot's joints), which signify loss of protective pain sensation (Fig. 6.1, p. 46).

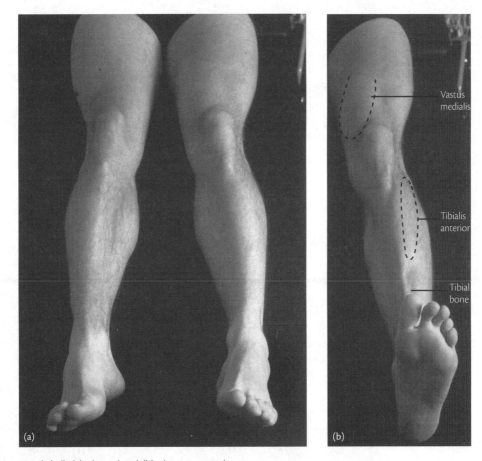

Fig. 2.31 Leg muscle bulk: (a) when relaxed; (b) when contracted.

Tone

The spasticity of an upper motor neuron lesion, best observed as clonus, is the most reliable tone change detectable in the legs. Elicit **ankle clonus** by externally rotating the foot and holding the knee slightly flexed with one hand, whilst sharply jerking the sole of the foot upwards with the other hand (Fig. 2.32). The foot should be held firmly in sustained dorsiflexion for a moment or two since the rhythmic downward beatings of clonus takes time to become evident. Sustained clonus, or un-sustained clonus of more than six beats, provides definite evidence of an upper motor neuron lesion.

Power

One proximal and one distal muscle should be tested to detect myopathy (proximal weakness) or peripheral neuropathy (distal weakness) or upper motor neuron lesions (both proximal and distal).

Hip flexion (iliopsoas muscle; L1, L2 roots) is tested by instructing the patient to 'push your leg up to 45°, and then pressing downwards just above the knee (Fig. 2.33).

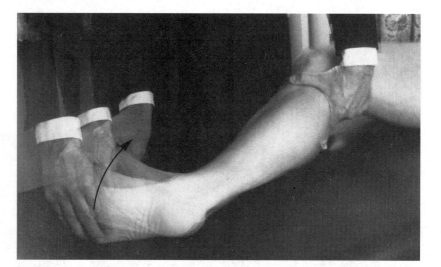

Fig. 2.32 Testing for ankle clonus.

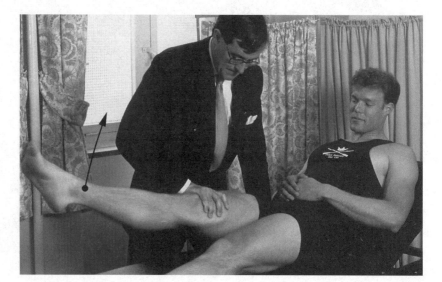

Fig. 2.33 Testing hip flexion power (iliopsoas).

Tibialis anterior (peroneal nerve; L5 root) can be tested by asking the patient to 'cock your foot up towards you' and then trying to overcome this (Fig. 2.34). It is particularly valuable to test tibialis anterior, since it will be weak in upper motor neuron lesions, in polyneuropathy, in common peroneal nerve lesions, and in L5/S1 root lesions due to prolapsed intervertebral disc.

Some leg muscles are so powerful that mild degrees of weakness cannot be detected reliably by bedside testing. For instance, knee extension by quadriceps (femoral nerve; L3, L4 roots) is best tested by asking a patient to stand up from a chair without using the arms. Ankle plantar flexion by gastrocnemius (posterior tibial nerve; S1, S2 roots) is best tested by asking a patient to stand on tiptoe or to hop.

Tendon reflexes

The **knee jerk** or **quadriceps tendon reflex** (femoral nerve; L3, L4 roots) is best tested by flexing both knees by 60–90°, and striking the patellar tendon (Fig. 2.35).

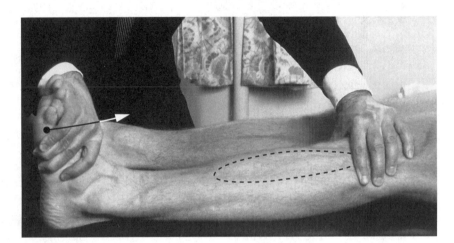

Fig. 2.34 Testing ankle dorsiflexion power (tibialis anterior).

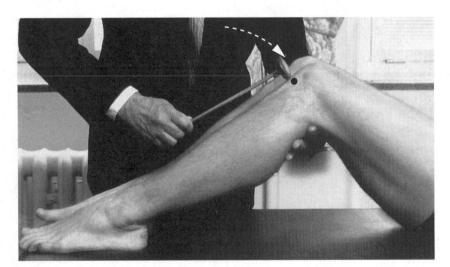

Fig. 2.35 Eliciting the knee jerk (L3/L4).

The **ankle jerk** or **gastrocnemius tendon reflex** (posterior tibial nerve; S1, S2 roots) is elicited by externally rotating one foot with the knee slightly bent, gently dorsiflexing the knee with the left hand, and then striking the Achilles tendon firmly with the hammer (Fig. 2.36). The ankle jerks are absent in many people over the age of 65. Inexperienced examiners are frequently unable to elicit the ankle jerks because they do not strike the Achilles tendon sufficiently firmly, or because the patient is rigidly holding their foot in dorsiflexion.

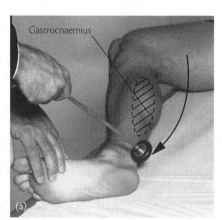

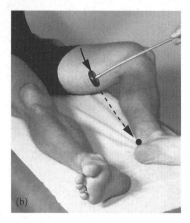

Fig. 2.36 Eliciting the ankle jerk (S1/S2).

Brisk reflexes point to an upper motor neuron lesion in which case-sustained ankle clonus and/or an extensor plantar response would be expected too. However, sometimes only one of this triad is present in upper motor neuron lesions. Slightly brisk reflexes may occur in anxious, tense patients. As with the arm reflexes, **reinforcement** should be undertaken before finally declaring a reflex absent.

Plantar responses

An **extensor** plantar or **Babinski** response is a definite sign of an upper motor neuron lesion. It is present immediately the lesion has occurred, well before the development of sufficient spasticity to allow clonus or hyperreflexia. Technique is all important for eliciting this reflex reliably. The patient should be lying down unable to see their toes. The examiner should passively wiggle the great toe up and down beforehand, both to ensure that it is relaxed, and also to detect hallux rigidis, which would mask an otherwise extensor response. Then, whilst lightly holding the leg just above the ankle with your left hand, hold a thin stick, your thumb nail, or a key in the right hand and slowly but firmly draw it up the outer aspect of the sole and across the ball of the foot (Fig. 2.37).

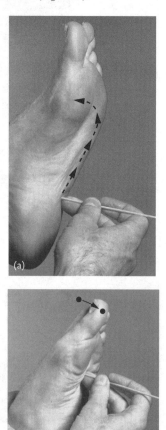

Fig. 2.37 (a) Eliciting the plantar response. (b) A flexor (normal) plantar response.

All the while you should watch the great toe from the side so as to detect whether its first movement is downwards (flexor and normal) (Fig. 2.37b) or upwards (extensor and abnormal) (Fig. 2.38).

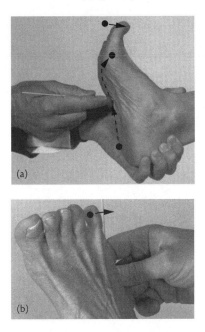

Fig. 2.38 An extensor plantar response with (a) dorsiflexion of the great toe and (b) fanning of the little toe.

Sensory examination

In a patient without sensory symptoms, such as deadness or tinglings, and whose Romberg test is normal, sensory examination is rarely abnormal. It is not worth performing as a routine if you do not suspect disease of the sensory pathways.

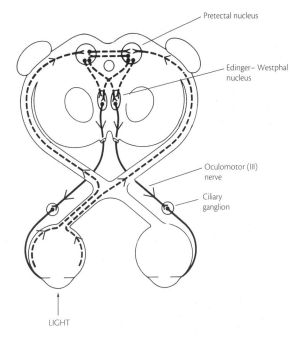

Fig. 2.39 Schematic circuitry for the 'unilateral afferent–bilateral efferent' reflexes illustrated by the pupil–light reflex mediated by the midbrain. The corneal and gag reflexes employ similar circuitry although innervate voluntary muscle.

Unilateral afferent–bilateral efferent reflexes

In this group of cranial reflexes a unilateral sensory stimulus evokes a bilateral motor response. An example of the circuitry is shown in Fig. 2.39 and should be memorized to interpret the effects of lesions affecting the afferent and efferent pathway(s) or the brain stem nucleus.

The reflexes obeying this circuitry are shown in Table 2.2.

TABLE 2.2 Unilateral afferent–bilateral efferent reflexes		
	Sensory stimulus (unilateral)	Motor response (bilateral)
Pupil–light reflex	Retinal illumination (optic nerve II)	Pupil constriction (oculomotor nerve III)
Blink reflex	Corneal touch (trigeminal nerve V)	Blinking (facial nerve VII)
Gag reflex	Palatal touch (glossopharyngeal nerve IX)	Soft palate elevation (vagus nerve X)

CHAPTER 3

Adding to the basic neurological examination

The following examples show how you should **add to the basic neurological examination** if the patient's symptoms suggest a specific disorder, if the basic examination throws up abnormalities requiring further evaluation, or if you are asked to examine a particular feature during an examination. Further details and other examples are given in other chapters.

Cranial nerves

You will have noted that the basic neurological examination in Chapter 2 does not test each cranial nerve in detail. You should know which main functions of each cranial nerve are easily testable, should the clinical situation require it.

I   **Olfactory nerve**. Test smell in each nostril with the eyes closed. See Chapter 17.

II **Optic nerve**. Optic fundi, visual acuity; fields; pupil–light response (afferent). See Chapters 2 and 14.

III **Oculomotor nerve**. Eye movements (horizontal adduction, up, down), eyelids; pupil–light response (efferent). See Chapter 14.

IV **Trochlear nerve**. Eye movement (down and in) 'look towards the tip of your nose'. See Chapter 14.

V   **Trigeminal nerve**. Jaw closure (masseter and temporalis); jaw opening (pterygoids); facial sensation;

corneal reflex (afferent) using wisp of cotton wool. See Chapter 2.

VI   **Abducens**. Eye movement (horizontal abduction). See Chapter 14.

VII   **Facial**. Facial muscles (test mouth and forehead); corneal reflex (efferent). See Chapters 2 and 13.

VIII **Auditory**. Hearing a whisper; Weber's and Rinne's tests with 512 Hz tuning fork. See Chapter 15.

IX   **Glossopharyngeal**. Use an orange stick to test palatal sensation and the gag reflex (afferent). See Chapters 2 and 13.

X   **Vagus**. Palatal movement; gag reflex (efferent); vocal cord movement (speaking, sharp cough). See Chapters 13 and 23.

XI   **(Spinal) accessory**. Shoulder shrugging and scapular rotation to abduction of the arm beyond 90° (trapezius; Fig. 3.8); head rotation laterally (sternomastoid).

XII   **Hypoglossal**. Tongue protrusion. See Chapters 2 and 13.

A weak, areflexic, or numb limb

(see Chapter 9)

A wide range of muscles and sensory territories must be examined using a strategy to distinguish between **root lesions, polyneuropathy, mononeuropathy, and myopathy**. For example, if a patient has weakness of the first dorsal interosseous muscle (ulnar nerve, T1 root; see Chapter 2), but abductor policis brevis (median nerve, also T1; see Chapter 10) remains strong, it is clear that there is an ulnar nerve lesion not a polyneuropathy or a T1 root lesion. Often you can compare the strength of a particular muscle in the patient with that of your own.

Other useful muscles to test in the arm

- **Supraspinatus** (shoulder abduction (0–15°), suprascapular nerve, C5 root);
- **Deltoid** (shoulder abduction (15–90°) axillary nerve, C5 root; see Fig. 2.25);
- **Biceps** (elbow flexion, musculocutaneous nerve, C5/C6 root; see Fig. 3.1);
- **Triceps** (elbow extension, radial nerve, C7/C8; Fig. 3.2);
- **Finger extensors** (radial/posterior interosseous nerve, C7; Fig. 3.3);
- **Flexor digitorum profundus** (terminal interphalangeal joint flexion, anterior interosseous branch of median nerve (index finger) or ulnar nerve (little finger, C7/C8); Fig. 3.4);
- **Dorsal interosseous** (ulnar nerve, T1; see Fig. 2.26).

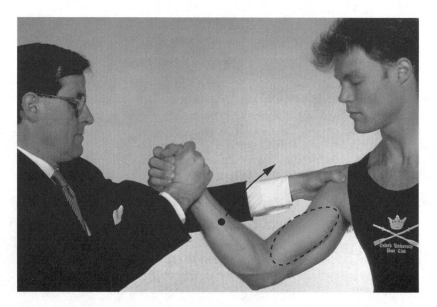

Fig. 3.1 Testing biceps power. Compare elbow flexion using your own biceps muscle to test the patient's biceps muscle. Stabilize the patient's shoulder with your other hand to prevent the trunk muscles from participating in the patient's pulling action.

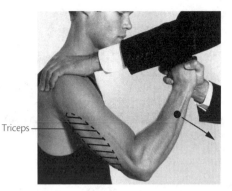

Triceps

Fig. 3.2 Testing triceps power. Test elbow extension using your own triceps muscle against the patient's triceps muscle. Stabilize the shoulder with your other hand to prevent the shoulder girdle muscles from participating in the pushing action.

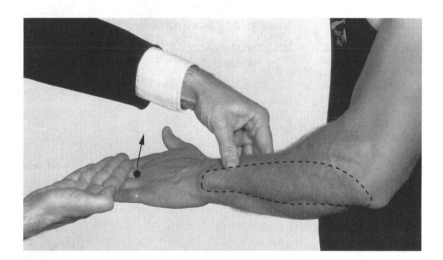

Fig. 3.3 Testing extensor digitorum power. Test finger extension using your own extended fingers for comparison.

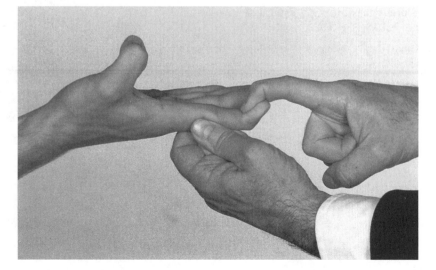

Fig. 3.4 Testing flexor digitorum profundus power. Compare the power of flexion at the distal interphalangeal joint by pulling against the patient's finger.

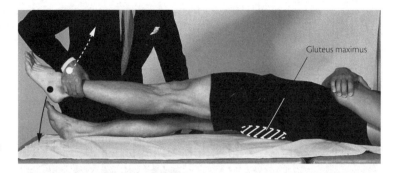

Fig. 3.5 Testing gluteus maximus power. Ask the patient to 'push your leg down into the couch' whilst you pull up on ankle. If the power is normal you can lift the patient's bottom off the couch.

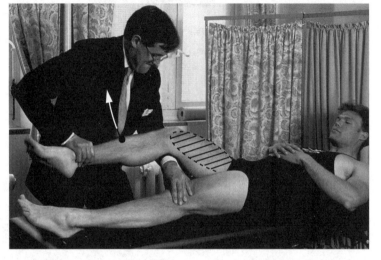

Fig. 3.6 Testing quadriceps power. Ask the patient to 'kick your leg out straight' whilst you push downwards on the ankle. This is a very powerful movement and it helps to put your left arm behind the knee, both to act as a fulcrum and to prevent hip extension from participating in the movement.

Useful muscles to test in the leg

- **Iliopsoas** (innervated by lumbar plexus, L1/L2 roots; see Fig. 2.33);

- **Gluteus maximus** (hip extension, Inferior gluteal nerve, L5/S1; Fig. 3.5);

- **Quadriceps** (knee extension, femoral nerve, L3/L4; Fig. 3.6);

- **Gastrocnemius** (ankle plantar flexion, tibial nerve, S1/S2; Fig. 3.7).

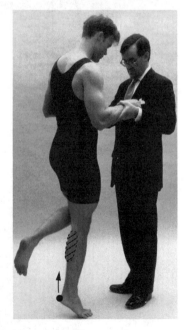

Fig. 3.7 Testing gastrocnemius power. A very strong muscle which is best tested by asking the patient to stand on tiptoe, or even to hop, whilst you steady him by holding his forearms.

Speech disorders (see Chapter 23)

In **dysphonia** the voice is quiet because the larynx produces sound inefficiently. The cough is 'bovine' without the normal sharp explosive onset allowed by suddenly opening a closed larynx.

Dysarthria is an inability to shape noise into recognizable words. Slurred and slow pronunciation is obvious on repeating words with lots of consonants, such as 'uNiVeRSiTy' or 'WeST ReGiSTeR STReeT' or 'ePiSCoPaL CoNSTiTuTioN'.

Dysphasias involve abnormalities in the understanding of, or the generation of, language. Patients with a **receptive**, **Wernicke**, or **sensory dysphasia** are unable to understand and execute a simple three-stage command such as 'When I clap my hands, please touch your right ear with your left index finger'. A **motor** or **Broca's dysphasia** causes a slowed rate of word production and word-finding difficulties.

Dementia (see Chapter 24)

Dementia is a diffuse loss of cognitive function. Check **orientation** for time and date, place and person. Test **calculation** by serial subtraction of 7 from 100. Is **general knowledge** consistent with the patient's background? Test **memory** by immediate and 5-minute recall of a simple three line address or of three objects. **Cognitive estimates** such as 'Roughly how long is a man's spine?' or 'How many camels are there in Holland?' may be abnormal in frontal lobe disease. Observe the patient's demeanour for the flat or gloomy affect typical of **depression**; this may be a clue to pseudodementia. Look for the poor grooming and self-neglect, or the failure to use gesture and vacant facial expression reflecting **loss of non-verbal communication** as occurs in global dementia. Test **right parietal lobe spatial functions** by asking the patient to draw or copy a three-dimensional cube. Or, if dysphasia prevents understanding of this instruction, look for dressing apraxia by seeing whether the patient can put on a garment correctly when it has one sleeve pulled through the wrong way.

Abnormal sphincter control

In a patient with hesitancy of micturition, retention, or incontinence of urine, you need to test the **plantar responses** to detect a spinal cord lesion affecting the upper motor neurons, and the **ankle jerks** and **perianal pinprick sensation** to detect cauda equina compression or peripheral neuropathy. Indeed these three tests are the entire neurological examination required in the urology clinic to screen patients with apparent prostatism for a contributory neurological disorder.

Stroke (see Chapter 27)

Cardiovascular examination is often more pertinent than neurological examination in cerebrovascular disease. It is essential to examine the **pulse** for arrhythmia, and the **blood pressure** for hypertension. Listen for **heart murmurs** indicating valvar disease and to the **carotid arteries** for the bruit of a stenosis; either may be the source of cerebral emboli.

Systemic tumours

If a focal neurological abnormality of the brain, spinal cord, or nerve roots suggests compression or infiltration by tumour, look for a primary tumour by examining all lymph node groups, the breasts, testicles, chest (including a radiograph), abdomen, rectum, and prostate or vagina.

Sciatica (see Chapter 9)

The **back** must be examined for focal tenderness which might indicate a vertebral tumour deposit. **Straight leg raising** will be unilaterally restricted to less than 80–90° in prolapsed intervertebral disc affecting the L5 or S1 nerve roots. Muscles innervated by the different nerve roots under suspicion should be tested, particularly ankle dorsiflexion (L5/S1). Pinprick sensation in the relevant dermatomes should be compared on the two sides.

Suspected Parkinson's disease (see Chapter 26)

Observe the patient during history taking for **paucity of facial expression** or a **pill-rolling rest tremor** of the finger and thumb. Observe the **gait** for a slow and shuffling start, or **loss of arm swing**. Unilateral **loss of arm swing** whilst walking may be the earliest sign. Look for **cog-wheel rigidity** of the arms. Does the patient have **micrographia** (Fig. 26.2) in which the letters get smaller during the writing of a word?

Coma (see Chapter 22)

An unconscious patient cannot cooperate with the usual examination. **General examination** will reveal cardiovascular shock, arrhythmia, a respiratory crisis, pyrexia, alcohol intoxication, head trauma, or the pinpoint pupils of opiate overdose. Blood sugar testing will reveal hypo- or hyperglycaemia. **Neck stiffness** will indicate meningism due to subarachnoid haemorrhage or meningitis. Regular spontaneous **breathing** may be lost in severe damage to brainstem respiratory nuclei. Cheyne–Stokes respiration (irregular waxing and waning) may indicate a forebrain lesion.

A **decerebrate posture** with the limbs stiffly extended usually indicates a brainstem lesion. The depth of unconsciousness is reflected by the extent of any **withdrawal response** to painful squeezing of the fingernails or toenails. If withdrawal is more severely affected on one side, this may indicate a contralateral cerebral lesion. The plantar responses are often extensor in unconscious patients and have little specific diagnostic value.

Brainstem function can be tested by eliciting:

- the **vestibulo-ocular reflex** of compensatory eye movements in response to head rotation or cold water irrigation of the ears;

- the **corneal response** of eye closure to cotton wool;

- the **cough** or **gag responses** to pharyngeal stimulation with a stick or sucker.

Some or all of these will be absent in brainstem disease.

CASE 3.1 'A MISERABLE END: CANCER IN THE SKULL BASE'

A 40-year-old man had received full-dose radiotherapy and extensive chemotherapy for a pharyngeal lymphoma. Nine months later he developed steadily worsening aching pain deeply located seemingly in the skull near his right ear. Then he developed spasms of pain radiating to the back of his throat on the right. The gag reflex was not elicitable from stroking the right palate. As if this combination of bony ache and neuralgic pains were not enough, the misery of his condition intensified when he started inhaling drinking fluids and developed a quiet, inefficient, dysphonic voice. A bovine cough showed he had weakness of vocal cord closure due to laryngeal nerve fibre involvement. The right side of his palate did not elevate either voluntarily or to gag reflex testing; this showed that the laryngeal weakness was due to a lesion of the parent trunk of the vagus nerve rather than a more peripheral lesion of the laryngeal nerve branches. When viewed from behind there was wasting of his right trapezius muscle and he was unable to use this muscle to rotate the shoulder blade so as to raise his arm above his head (Fig. 3.8).

CT scan of the skull base showed a deposit of lymphoma in the region of the jugular foramen, through which the glossopharyngeal (IX), vagus (X), and accessory (XI) nerves run (Fig. 3.9). Further chemotherapy did not prevent progression. No more radiotherapy could be given without likely damage to the spinal cord or brainstem. Such infiltrating lesions are not amenable to surgery. This brave man remained stoical until his end came from inhalational pneumonia, his pain having required opiate analgesia.

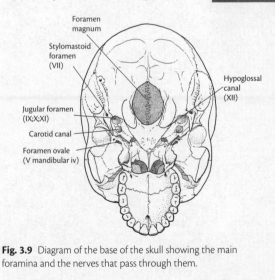

Wasted right trapezius

Fig. 3.8 The accessory nerve lesion showing: (a) wasting of the right trapezius muscle; and (b) inability to abduct the arm beyond 90°.

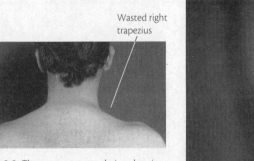

Foramen magnum
Stylomastoid foramen (VII)
Jugular foramen (IX;X;XI)
Carotid canal
Foramen ovale (V mandibular iv)
Hypoglossal canal (XII)

Fig. 3.9 Diagram of the base of the skull showing the main foramina and the nerves that pass through them.

Comment

◆ Malignant bone pain, nerve infiltration pain, and choking are all horrible afflictions. When combined in skull base malignancy the overall effect can be truly miserable.

◆ From a diagnostic point of view, this constellation of cranial nerve abnormalities enabled the anatomical location of the lesion to be predicted quite precisely (Fig. 3.9). The diagnosis was proved by directing detailed CT scanning with bone window settings of the skull base.

CHAPTER 4

Neurology in children and the elderly

The conventional approach to neurology relates primarily to assessment of patients between the ages of about 10 and 70. Other methods must be used to obtain a history and examine younger children, and to define what is neurologically abnormal in the elderly.

Children

The parents

Very often it is the parents who are more concerned than their child about the possibility of neurological disease. Neurological evaluation is easiest in a child-friendly environment. Indeed much of the child's ability to comply with a neurological examination reflects their own parents' confidence in the doctor, and in the clinical environment.

History

Children, especially when very young, cannot respond as specifically as adults to detailed questions about their symptoms, and especially their time course. Children find it particularly hard to give meaningful accounts of sensory symptoms or pain. Young children are often surprisingly undisturbed by serious negative symptoms involving loss of functions such as vision.

Although it is important for the parent to summarize the history and its time course, you should always try to obtain the child's own version, however, rudimentary. Sometimes the dynamics of the family situation may make the clinical consultation difficult. Parents may be troubled by overwhelming anxiety or guilt, particularly if there is a question of familial disease. Parents may underestimate their child's disabilities, either because they do not have other children against whom to compare development, or because of an optimistically dissonant attitude to their child's difficulties. Rarely, but importantly, a parent may fabricate aspects of the child's illness, and invent plausible explanations, possibly to divert attention from abuse or violence.

The antenatal and birth history is important, particularly in children with intellectual or motor developmental delay. Antenatally, a maternal history of alcoholism or of infections such as rubella, cytomegalovirus, syphilis, HIV, or toxoplasmosis can cause brain damage; such infections may have been subclinical in the mother. Medicinal or recreational drugs consumed during pregnancy should be checked for their potential to cause congenital damage. Preterm delivery, especially if associated with low birth weight, predisposes to neurological disorders, particularly cerebral palsy. Abnormalities of delivery can cause ischaemic brain damage.

Developmental milestones

Cerebral palsy consists of delayed motor development due to damage to the developing brain. It is non-progressive and with normal or near normal underlying intellect. By contrast, children with cognitive impairments are backward in all aspects of development, with varying involvement of motor functions. Some fail to develop close emotional bonds with their mother. Children with generalized cognitive impairments are at particular risk of epilepsy, and additional behavioural disturbances including attention-deficit hyperactivity disorder, the autistic spectrum of disorders, persisting immaturities of behaviour such as slobbering and putting things in their mouth, and development of stereotypies such as repetitive rocking and vocalizations.

The mother should be asked when the child mastered certain skills. The following milestones are easy to remember:

- Were fetal movements normal?
- 1–2 months: social smiling
- 4 months: head control while sitting supported
- 6 months: starts sitting unaided
- 10–16 months: walks
- 15 months: a few words in addition to 'mum' and 'dad'
- 2 years: simple sentences
- 3–4 years: uses lavatory
- 5 years: dresses independently.

Neurological examination

Beyond the age of 5, a relaxed child can be examined in much the same way as an adult. It helps to keep the examination as short as possible to maintain concentration. Tendon reflexes are particularly difficult if the child is reluctant to stay still, or tends to stiffen or withdraw at the prospect of a tendon hammer blow. Children may be reassured by the charade of seeing reflexes elicited in their parent, or on a doll. Sensory testing is particularly difficult in those below 10 years of age.

In young children, particularly below the age of 5, a more informal approach should be taken to examination. Specific examination features, such as tendon reflexes are best conducted with the child sitting in the parent's lap. Vision, muscle power, and coordination are best assessed by watching the child run around, and play with bricks and beads.

Because of the subtle changes with age, language and cognitive function may require specialist assessment if important for diagnosis or planning education. Cerebral dominance can be deduced by observing writing, throwing, and kicking. Handedness normally does not appear before 2 years; clear hand preference before this age should make you suspect mild hemiparesis.

Assessing infants is particularly difficult. By 3 months, an infant should be able to follow with his eyes, by 7 months to transfer objects from hand to hand, and by 10 months to pick up small objects using finger–thumb opposition. By 3–4 months good head control should appear when the child is sitting or is pulled up from the lying position. The plantar responses are extensor until about 1 year of age.

If there is a question of hydrocephalus, head circumference can be plotted against standard values. The posterior fontanelle normally closes by 6 weeks of age, and the anterior by 10–20 months. Foot deformity and urinary incontinence should provoke a search for spina bifida. Children with epilepsy may have tuberous sclerosis and skin examination may reveal unpigmented patches, the spots of epiloia on the cheeks, or periungual fibromas at the nail edges.

The elderly

Spectrum of disorders

Many of those presenting with disabling neurological diseases are elderly; stroke, Parkinson's disease, dementia, and cervical spondylitic myelopathy being common. Troublesome neurological symptoms evading formal diagnosis are common in older patients. Examples include mild degrees of memory difficulty, dizziness, and falls of uncertain cause, or undiagnosable blackouts and funny turns. Gait disorders are particularly common in the very old, usually consisting of small steps and difficulty in turning corners. In elderly patients, particular effort should be made to pursue diagnoses which may lead to improvement or stabilization of a disorder during the patient's natural lifespan. Examples include subdural haematoma, meningioma, Parkinson's disease, herpes encephalitis, hydrocephalus, idiopathic demyelinating polyneuropathy, lumbar spinal canal stenosis, and myasthenia gravis.

Neurological examination becomes less discriminating in older patients

Absent ankle jerks, loss of vibration sense from the feet, mild weakness of ankle dorsiflexion, and generalized reduction in muscle bulk are frequent findings in patients over 65. They only assume clear pathological significance if unilateral, or if they have been observed to emerge at a rapid rate during sequential examinations. Small pupils and loss of upgaze are frequent asymptomatic ocular signs. Hearing, smell, and taste all deteriorate with ageing. By the age of 80, almost everyone's gait shows small strides, uncertainty, disequilibrium, a widened base, use of a stick, and difficulty with sharp cornering. Heel–toe walking is often impossible for elderly patients without there being any clearly identifiable ataxic process.

CHAPTER 5

A general introduction to muscular weakness

In a patient with muscular weakness, simple clinical assessment will usually localize the anatomical level of the lesion (Fig. 5.1) to one of the following:

♦ the upper motor neuron,

♦ the lower motor neuron,

♦ the peripheral nerve,

♦ the muscle itself.

You should be familiar with the descriptive terminology of limb weakness. Weakness of one limb is often called **monoparesis**, complete paralysis being termed monoplegia. Weakness of both legs is **paraparesis** or paraplegia if complete. Weakness of the arm and leg on one side only is known as **hemiparesis** or hemiplegia. Weakness of all four limbs is termed either **tetraparesis** or quadriparesis (tetraplegia or quadriplegia).

These terms describe the pattern of weakness but do not imply any localization of the responsible lesion.

When testing muscle power, a few general principles help. First, make the patient's task clear both by your words and the way you place your hands. Second whenever possible use your own muscle to test the identical muscle in the patient's arm—this makes the test sensitive to minor degrees of weakness. Third, the physique of doctors and patients varies and you should develop sensitive ways of testing muscle power that suit and match your physical abilities. Fourth, use one hand to prevent unwanted movements from occurring. For instance, to prevent trunk rotation during biceps testing, a mere touch on the shoulder will suffice to inhibit movement; forcible restraint of the patient's shoulder is unnecessary.

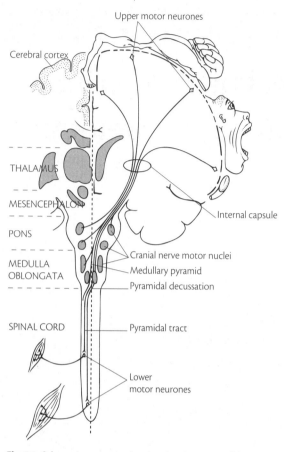

Fig. 5.1 Schematic representation showing the course of the pyramidal tract, the homuncular organization of the motor cortex in the precentral gyrus, the concentration of the motor output within the internal capsule, the decussation of the pyramidal tract in the medulla oblongata, and the synaptic connections with lower motor neuron pools in the spinal cord and brainstem.

Upper motor neuron lesions

Upper motor neuron lesions can arise either in the spinal cord or in the brain. In **spinal cord lesions**, the weakness is usually bilateral causing paraparesis or tetraparesis (arms and legs). **Brain lesions** usually affect only one cerebral hemisphere, so the weakness is usually a contralateral hemiparesis which often includes the face. Although skin sensation is affected in most spinal cord lesions, that is not usually the case for brain lesions.

The incontrovertible physical sign of upper motor neuron damage is the **extensor plantar response** (Babinski response; Fig. 2.38). Once an upper motor neuron lesion has been present for a fortnight or so, the limb tone becomes spastic with a **pronator catch** in the arm

(Fig. 2.23) or sustained **ankle clonus** (Fig. 2.32), and brisk **tendon reflexes**. However, in the first few days after an acute upper motor neuron lesion, such as a cerebral hemisphere stroke or a traumatic spinal cord lesion, the tone remains flaccid and the reflexes may be absent, although the plantar response becomes extensor immediately. Severe upper motor neuron lesions cause complete paralysis of the affected limbs. Milder lesions cause a pattern of weakness which characteristically predominates in the antigravity muscles of the leg (hip and knee flexors, ankle dorsiflexors) and in the shoulder abductors, and elbow and finger extensors of the arm.

Lower motor neuron damage

Damage to lower motor neurons may occur in **peripheral nerve** or **nerve root lesions** or as part of the diffuse neurodegenerative disorder known as **motor neuron disease**. The pattern of muscle involvement reflects which of these structures is affected and in which part of the body. Skin sensory loss usually accompanies peripheral nerve lesions. Patients with single nerve root lesions often have sensory symptoms, such as pain or tingling, but demonstrable sensory loss is not so usual. Patients with motor neuron diseases have no sensory symptoms or loss.

Wasting, fasciculations, and areflexia are the common features of lower motor neuron lesions.

Wasting

Wasting develops in any muscle that has been significantly denervated for more than 4–6 weeks. This wasting will be restricted to those muscles supplied by the affected nerve root or peripheral nerve. In axonal degeneration polyneuropathy only the distal limb muscles will be symmetrically weak and wasted because it predominantly affects long axons. In motor neuron diseases which affect the neuron cell body in the spinal cord, weakness and wasting are usually both proximal and distal, and may be asymmetric.

Fasciculations

Fasciculations occur during subacute partial denervation of muscles, and are a particularly common feature of motor neuron disease. A fasciculation is a momentarily flickering contraction which is visible within the belly of a muscle. It represents simultaneous contraction of all the muscle fibres in the motor unit innervated by a single motor neuron (Fig. 5.2).

Fasciculations are most easily visualized in those muscles with large motor units each containing hun-

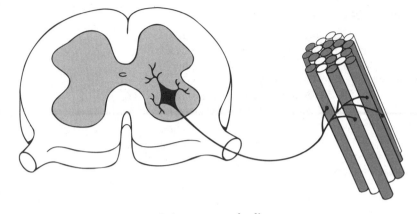

Fig. 5.2 A single motor neuron innervating a motor unit of muscle fibres, interspersed with the muscle fibres of other motor units. A fasciculation is a simultaneous contraction of all the muscle fibres in a single motor unit.

dreds of muscle fibres, such as powerful proximal limb muscles. They are not easily seen in those muscles with small motor units which are used for fine motor control, such as the small hand muscles. However, electromyographic examination will detect fasciculations in any denervated muscle, large or small.

Areflexia

Loss of tendon reflexes is common in lower motor neuron lesions. However, this is mainly because of coexisting involvement of the muscle spindle sensory afferent fibres within peripheral nerves or roots (Fig. 5.3). The tendon reflexes are preserved late into motor neuron disease until the muscle is severely denervated, because in that disease the sensory afferents are not affected.

Primary muscle disease

In weakness due to primary muscle disease, there is never any sensory loss. As a general rule, the weakness affects mainly the **proximal limb muscles** in acquired muscle diseases, such as inflammatory or metabolic myopathies. However, the pattern of weakness and wasting varies and can pick out specific muscle groups in certain muscular dystrophies. Normally the tendon reflexes are retained in muscle disease.

Wasting is variably present in muscle disease. Most muscular dystrophies and inflammatory myopathies cause wasting of the affected muscles. In the severe sex-linked recessive muscular dystrophy of Duchenne, hypertrophy (often known as pseudohypertrophy) affects the weakened calf muscle. In myasthenia gravis, a disorder of neuromuscular transmission, the muscles are not wasted, and the weakness gets worse with use: so-called fatigability.

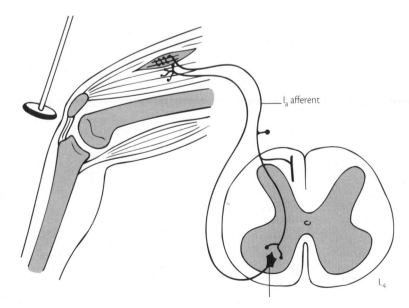

I$_a$ afferent

L$_4$

Fig. 5.3 The components of the monosynaptic stretch reflex arc elicited by percussing the patellar tendon of the quadriceps muscle.

Distinctive patterns of weakness

Various forms of muscular dystrophy pick out specific groups of muscles which are often summarized by the diagnostic title: facioscapulo-humeral or oculopharyngeal dystrophies for example. Myasthenia gravis may present with either ptosis and eye movement disorders, or with pharyngeal and palatal weakness causing nasal regurgitation of drinking fluids, or with proximal limb weakness. Neck extensor muscle weakness is unusual, distinctively occurring in myasthenia gravis, motor neuron disease, myotonic dystrophy, and some myopathies.

Disuse atrophy

Generalized disuse atrophy of muscles occurs in patients who have been recumbent for general medical reasons. Focal disuse atrophy may affect muscles acting on a diseased joint such as the quadriceps muscle in knee joint disease. Disuse atrophy can be distinguished from the wasting due to lower motor neuron or muscle disease because the reflexes and tone are normal, and no fasciculations occur. But most importantly, strength is relatively well preserved in a disuse atrophied muscle, whereas a pathologically wasted muscle will be profoundly weakened.

Fluctuating weakness

Many patients demonstrate momentarily fluctuating, inconsistent, or collapsing patterns of weakness. This has three possible causes:

1 **Psychologically determined** weakness fluctuates and may be temporarily improved by encouragement. In more extreme cases there may be associated theatrical grunting and sighing in a charade of effort, and the collapsing may occur more from the trunk than the limb itself. The severity of limb strength during formal testing may be discordant with obviously better usage of the limb during natural activities such as dressing or walking, especially if these are seemingly unobserved.

2 **Pain** in a joint may be associated with complaint of discomfort. The raw power of the muscle can be assessed by 'push as hard as you can for just a moment when I count to three'.

3 **Sensory loss** affecting kinaesthetic feedback usually produces apparent muscle weakness affecting the hand, which is a complex motor–sensory organ. This is generally associated with pseudoathetosis (Fig. 2.28) in which the finger cannot maintain a constant position with the eyes closed. This type of weakness is usually improved by asking the patient to carry out the movement whilst watching their hand, thereby providing compensatory visual feedback.

Some patients seem to be unable to relax their legs during examination. To some degree this is common in otherwise normal elderly patients. If extreme, or occurring before old age, it can be a sign of frontal lobe disease, known as **gegenhalten** tone.

Summary

Table 5.1 summarizes the physical signs associated with the various causes of muscle weakness.

	Upper motor neuron damage		Lower motor neuron damage	Primary muscle disease	Psychogenic disorder
Sign	Cerebral hemisphere	Spinal cord			
Wasting			Present	Present	
Fasciculations			Present		
Reflexes	Brisk	Brisk	Absent	Normal	Normal
Tone	Spastic	Spastic	Flaccid	Normal	Normal
Plantars[a]	↑↓	↑↑	↓↓	↓↓	↓↓
Sensory loss	Sometimes	Usually	Usually	No	Often
Distribution of weakness	Hemiplegic	Paraplegic or quadriplegic	Individual peripheral nerve or root; distal in polyneuropathy	Proximal	Varies

TABLE 5.1 Physical signs in weakness: a summary

[a] ↑: extensor plantar response; ↓ : flexor plantar response.

CHAPTER 6

Patterns of sensory loss

Unlike the situation with muscle weakness, clinical examination is not nearly so effective for localizing the level in the nervous system of a lesion causing a somatosensory disturbance. Furthermore, meaningful examination of sensation is surprisingly difficult. However, this difficulty is due largely to poorly thought out strategy for presenting the test stimuli. This chapter will concentrate on the different approaches needed first to map out and interpret skin sensory loss and second to establish thresholds for joint position and vibration sensations.

Sensory symptoms

Sensory symptoms can be distinctive.

- **Parasthesiae**, or pins and needles, usually occur in acquired (not inherited) polyneuropathy or in com-

pressive lesions of individual peripheral nerves. Parasthesiae are less common in root lesions and intrinsic spinal cord disease.

- **Lancinating pain** radiating down a limb like electric shocks should suggest nerve root compression by prolapsed intervertebral disc, for example, sciatica.

- **Painless injuries** to digits, such as puncture injuries or burns, occur in peripheral neuropathies which predominantly damage the unmyelinated pain and temperature fibres. Examples include diabetic polyneuropathy, or diseases affecting the spinothalamic tracts within the spinal cord, such as syringomyelia (see Chapter 8). Similarly, loss of pain feedback can lead to joint disruption and degeneration, so-called **Charcot joints** (Fig. 6.1).

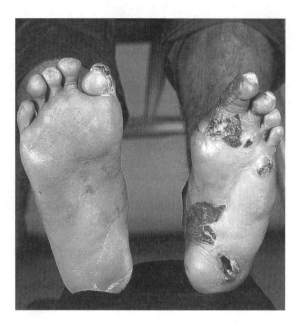

Fig. 6.1 Painless injuries to the foot in hereditary sensory neuropathy. Traumatic skin damage leading to chronic ulceration, Charcot joints, and autoamputation of a toe are all evident.

- **Gait unsteadiness** can be due to joint position sense loss in the feet. Patients may topple when they close their eyes in the shower or try to walk in the dark; this is **Rombergism** (Fig. 2.2, p. 7).

- **Astereognosis** occurs in patients with parietal lobe lesions. They cannot identify coins in their pocket or with their eyes closed.

- **Numbness** is a term that is used confusingly. Most doctors mean 'a loss of sensation', but many patients really mean weakness or clumsiness. It is less ambiguous to ask about 'deadness (or loss) of skin sensation'. Polyneuropathy produces numbness in a glove and stocking distribution. When patients describe numbness and/or pins or needles extending onto the trunk, it is most commonly due to myelitis,

an inflammation of the spinal cord, which may occur as part of multiple sclerosis.

Testing superficial sensation

To map the boundary of a patch of sensory loss you should start within the numb area and work outwards to the surrounding normal areas. Traditionally, an unused pin or a wisp of cotton wool are recommended. However, neither patients nor doctors are familiar with the thresholds for such sensations on different parts of the body. This makes it difficult to report whether the quality of sensation is altered, and it is rare for skin anaesthesia to be complete. However, patients are familiar with the feeling of fingertips on every part of their body skin and can instantly tell you whether the 'finger feels normal' when you stroke any patch of skin lightly. Furthermore, you can use both your forefingers to make a simultaneous comparison of the two sides of the patient's body or two adjacent patches of skin. Only rarely do you need to test temperature sensation; if so the cold metal of a tuning fork provides sufficient stimulus.

Patterns of skin sensory loss

Before you try and map out a patch of skin sensory disturbance you should think out a strategy to answer the clinical question facing you. Questions that commonly arise concern whether the patch of sensory disturbance has the typical distribution of:

- **an individual peripheral nerve territory or mononeuropathy** (Fig. 6.2);

- **an individual root lesion** (Fig 6.3);

- **polyneuropathy** (distal glove and stocking) (Fig. 6.4);

- **myelitis** (with numbness extending from a limb onto the trunk (Fig. 6.5);

- **a compressive spinal cord lesion** producing a 'sensory level' on the trunk (Fig 6.6).

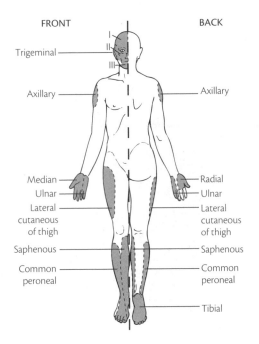

Fig. 6.2 Skin territories of some commonly damaged peripheral nerves.

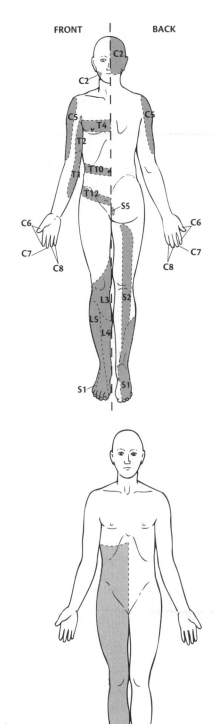

Fig. 6.3 Skin territories of landmark nerve roots.

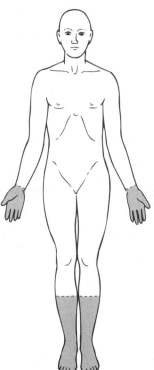

Fig. 6.4 Glove and stocking sensory loss in polyneuropathy.

Fig. 6.5 Sensory loss in myelitis. Of course, the distribution varies depending upon which part of the spinal cord is affected, and can be bilateral.

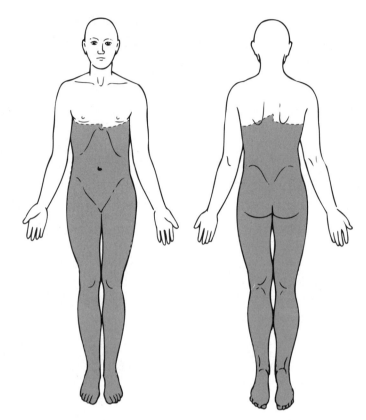

Fig. 6.6 A 'sensory level' in compression of the spinal cord at the T5 segment.

Practical psychophysics

Often it seems to be difficult to get consistent and meaningful information when testing perceptions such as joint position or visual fields. Usually this is due to poorly thought out strategy for testing which lacks objectivity. If you apply the psychophysical principles of **blinding**, **forced choice**, or **time-locking**, you can immediately make the following tests (Table 6.1) work reliably, as long as you have given the patient clear instructions.

1 **Blinding**. Close the patient's eyes so they cannot see when the stimulus changes.

2 **Forced choice**. Ask the patient to choose the direction of a stimulus. For example 'Tell me whether I move your toe up or down' or 'Point to the finger which moves' [one in each visual field].

TABLE 6.1	Using psychophysical principles to test perceptions		
	Blinding	Forced choice	Time-locking
Olfaction	YES		'Tell me WHEN you smell something' [as you bring the test smell slowly to the nostril].
Visual fields to confrontation		'Point to my finger[e.g. WHICH SIDE] when it moves'.	'Point to my finger WHEN it moves'.
Joint position sensation	YES	'Tell me whether your toe moves UP or DOWN'	
Vibration sensation	YES		'Tell me WHEN the tuning fork stops buzzing'.

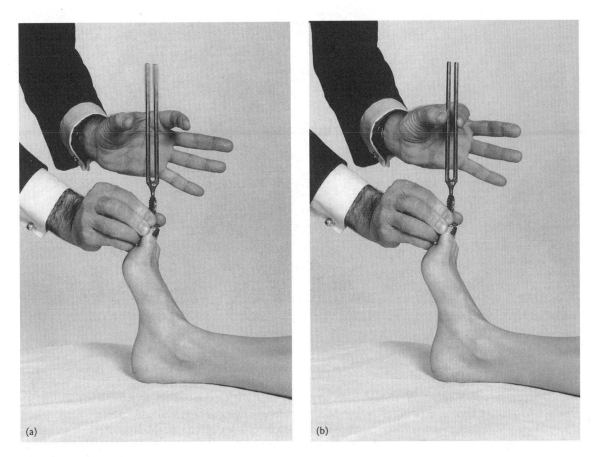

(a)   (b)

Fig. 6.7 Testing vibration sense. (a) The fingers of one hand are positioned ready to (b) stop the tuning fork vibrating and the patient is instructed to say 'now' when the tuning fork stops buzzing

3 **Time-locking**. Ask the patient to tell you *when* the stimulus changes. For example 'Point to my finger *when* it moves' or 'Tell me *when* the tuning fork stops buzzing' or 'Tell me *when* you smell something'.

Testing vibration sensation

For vibration sensation you should use a 128 Hz tuning fork and strike it in such a way that it does not produce audible high frequency harmonics which can be heard rather than felt by the patient. Place it on the patient's sternum and ask 'can you feel it buzzing?' Then move it to the tip of the great toe, or a finger, and ask the patient

to 'close your eyes, and tell me *when* it stops buzzing'. Then the patient should respond promptly when you stop the buzzing prongs with the fingers of your other hand (Fig. 6.7).

If vibration sense is absent from the toes you should work proximally along the ankle, tibial bone, knee, anterior superior iliac crest, and finally to the rib cage. Vibration sense abnormalities usually mean there is a polyneuropathy affecting large myelinated sensory fibres, or a spinal cord lesion. Vibration sense is not affected by a lesion restricted to the somatosensory cerebral cortex. Vibration sense is lost from the lower legs in many elderly people as a natural ageing phenomenon.

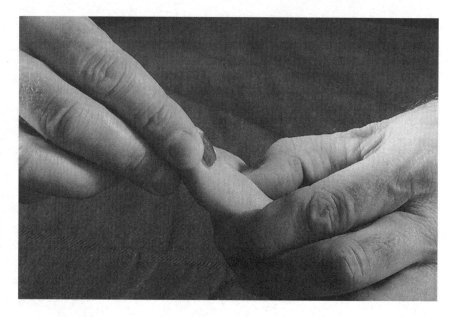

Fig. 6.8 Testing joint position sense at the great toe. The proximal phalanx is steadied with one hand whilst the toe is moved up or down

Testing joint position sense

With the patient's eyes open, you should move the great toe up and then down, showing the patient 'this is up (or down)'. Then ask the patient to close their eyes and identify small movements 'Tell me whether I move your toe *up* or *down*' (Fig. 6.8).

The distal interphalangeal joints of the fingers can be tested similarly. Normally people can identify tiny movements of a joint. Joint position sensation is lost in similar conditions to vibration sensation and is particularly likely to be abnormal in patients with sensory ataxia or Rombergism. But unlike vibration sensation, joint position perception is also lost in lesions of the somatosensory cortex.

CHAPTER 7

Weakness I: brain lesions

Clinical aspects

Hemiparesis

A lesion of one cerebral hemisphere produces hemiparesis on the opposite side with weakness affecting the leg, arm, and face. The two commonest causes are stroke, in which case the weakness comes on abruptly, or a tumour, which causes slow progression over weeks, months, or even years. Depending upon the exact site of the lesion within the cerebral hemisphere, the weakness may predominantly or solely affect either the face, arm, or leg. Any facial weakness affects only the mouth, but not the forehead muscles.

Hemiparesis arises due to lesions of the upper motor neurons at the level of the cell bodies of the precentral gyrus or of the axons passing through the internal capsule, cerebral peduncle, or brainstem. Lesions of the internal capsule are more likely to produce a complete hemiparesis whereas cortex lesions are more likely to pick out just a hand or a leg (a **monoparesis**) or the face (see Fig. 5.1, p. 42).

Cortical sensory loss

Cortical sensory loss due to cerebral hemisphere lesions is less frequently encountered than hemiparesis. Lesions affecting the somatosensory cerebral cortex posterior to the central sulcus impair **joint position** sense, reduce **two-point discrimination**, and cause **astereognosis** on the opposite side of the body. Lesions restricted to the adjacent parietal lobe produce **sensory inattention**. This can be tested by touching both sides of the patient simultaneously when their eyes are closed. The patient will ignore the stimulus contralateral to the side of the lesion, even though the touch is recognized if presented to that side alone.

Thalamic sensory loss

Unilateral loss of pain and temperature sensation can occur with lesions of the posterior thalamus. These are usually due to small infarcts. Chronic and intractable 'thalamic pain' syndromes can follow such lesions.

Brain scanning

CT (computed tomography) or MRI (magnetic resonance imaging) brain scans usually reveal the cause of hemiparesis or hemisensory disturbance. However, it should be noted that it may take a day or so for the typical appearances of a cerebral infarct to develop.

Computed tomography (CT) scanning

CT scanning uses X-rays. It is particularly good at detecting blood, which appears white due to its iron content. Calcification, such as the skull, also appears white. Increased water content appears black whether due to oedema or loss of normal brain tissue. White enhancement of vascular structures, and areas of blood–brain barrier breakdown due to inflammation or tumour, can be seen after intravenous injection of iodine-based contrast media (Fig. 7.1).

Magnetic resonance imaging (MRI)

MRI is much more sensitive than CT for imaging the substance of the brain and has replaced CT for most routine diagnostic work. It derives from the different radiofrequency signals produced by the protons of various tissue molecules which have been aligned by a powerful magnetic field and then displaced by radio-frequency pulses. MRI reveals the brainstem and cerebellum in much greater detail than CT because it is not degraded by the surrounding skull bones (Fig. 7.2). It is particularly useful for revealing demyelinating lesions in the brain and spinal cord white matter; these are generally invisible on CT. Intravenous gadolinium injection enhances vascular structures and areas of blood–brain barrier breakdown.

Interpreting brain scans

Armed with your knowledge of the gross anatomy of the brain you can detect most important abnormalities on scans by considering the following four aspects:

1 **Symmetry**. Do the two cerebral hemispheres look exactly the same? Or is there swelling on one side which displaces the midline, possibly due to a collection of blood outside the brain (Fig. 7.3), or a tumour or abscess within the brain and its surrounding oedema (Fig. 7.7).

2 Are there any **focal abnormalities** within the brain substance? Loss of normal tissue signal occurs in the plaques of demyelination (Fig. 7.4) or in the infarct of an ischaemic stroke (Fig. 7.5). The blood of an intracerebral haemorrhage (Fig. 7.6) or a tumour mass (Fig. 7.7) shows up well.

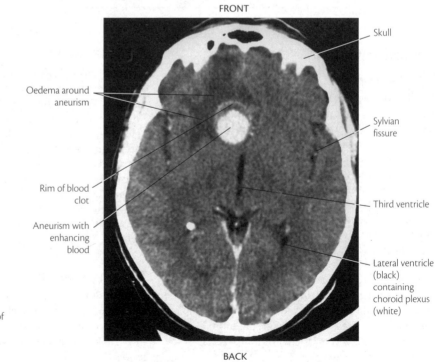

FRONT

Skull

Oedema around aneurism

Sylvian fissure

Rim of blood clot

Third ventricle

Aneurism with enhancing blood

Lateral ventricle (black) containing choroid plexus (white)

BACK

Fig. 7.1 A CT brain scan, contrast-enhanced, showing a giant suprasellar aneurism, full of blood with an anterior rim of blood clot, and some oedema of the adjacent cerebral hemisphere.

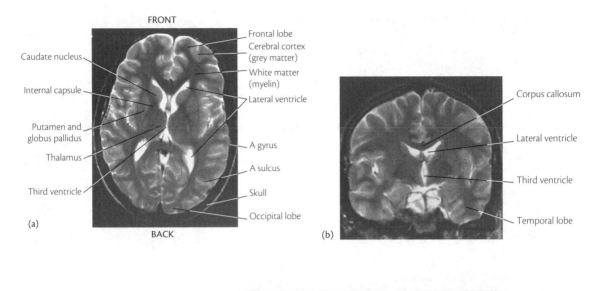

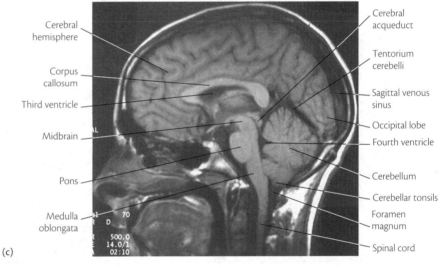

Fig. 7.2 Normal MRI.
(a) Horizontal section through cerebral hemispheres showing the major anatomical structures. (b) Coronal section through cerebral hemispheres. (c) Sagittal section through corpus callosum, cerebellum, and brainstem.

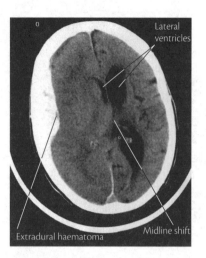

Fig. 7.3 Asymmetry of the brain, with midline shift due to an extradural haematoma (CT scan). Localized hydrocephalus is developing in the blocked lateral ventricles of the other hemisphere.

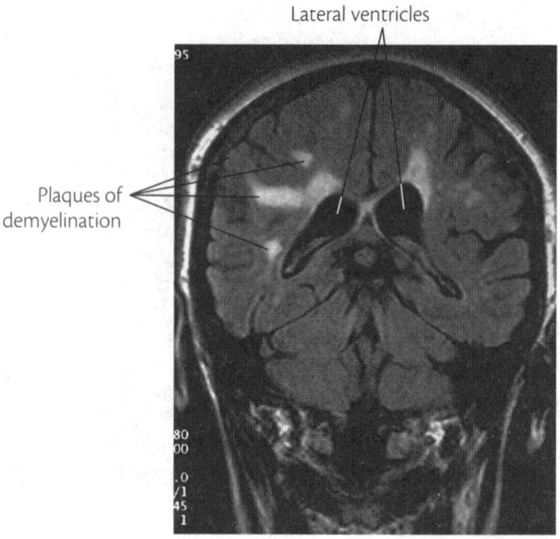

Fig. 7.4 Plaques of demyelination in the white matter adjacent to the lateral ventricles in a patient with multiple sclerosis (MRI, coronal section).

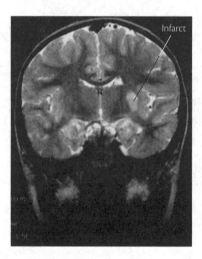

Fig. 7.5 A small infarct in the internal capsule/basal ganglia region (MRI, coronal section).

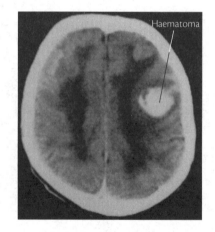

Fig. 7.6 An intracerebral haematoma (CT scan, unenhanced).

3 Are the **cerebral ventricles** distended by hydrocephalus? (Fig. 7.8).

4 Is there any abnormality **outside** the brain? Examples include focal collections of blood in a subdural or extradural haematoma (see Fig. 7.3), or a tumour of the meninges or skull (Fig. 7.9).

Brain tumours

The two commonest brain tumours in adults are **primary intracerebral gliomas** and **secondary deposits** from systemic tumours. Secondaries are usually derived from carcinomas of the breast, lung, gastrointestinal tract, or from melanoma. Primary cerebral **lymphomas** are increasingly common, especially in the elderly, and in those immunosuppressed by HIV infection or to prevent rejection of organ transplants. **Meningiomas** compress the brain from outside and are very slow growing (Fig. 7.9). Detection of a meningioma is especially important because it is the only tumour that can be completely and reliably removed neurosurgically. In adults most intrinsic brain tumours affect the cerebral hemi-

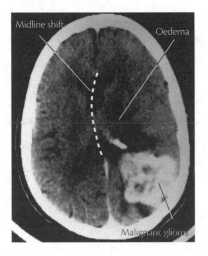

Fig. 7.7 A malignant glioma (CT scan, enhanced).

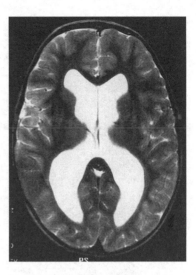

Fig. 7.8 The distended lateral and third ventricles of obstructive hydrocephalus (MRI scan).

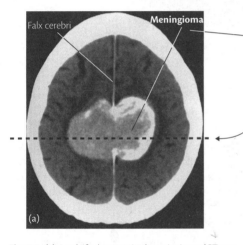

Fig. 7.9 (a) A calcified parasagittal meningioma (CT scan, unenhanced); (b) arising from the meninges of the falx cerebri above the brain and compressing the top of the motor cortex on both sides. This patient presented with bilateral leg weakness.

PARASAGITTAL MENINGIOMA

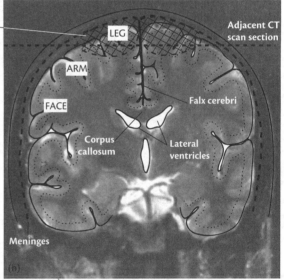

spheres. But in children it is the cerebellum that is usually affected by tumours such as **medulloblastoma** or **ependymoma** of the IVth ventricle.

Symptoms develop at different rates depending upon whether the tumour is malignant and rapidly growing; whether the tumour causes much surrounding oedema; and whether the tumour is affecting a 'noisy' part of the brain such as the motor cortex or cerebellar hemisphere instead of a relatively 'silent' part of the brain such as the frontal lobe. Common symptoms of

focal brain dysfunction are:

◆ homonymous hemianopia (occipital lobe);

◆ hemiplegia (contralateral motor cortex);

◆ disinhibition and lack of judgement (frontal lobe);

◆ dysphasia (left frontoparietal);

◆ unilateral ataxia (ipsilateral cerebellar hemisphere).

Focal or secondarily generalized **epilepsies** commonly result from tumours affecting the cerebral hemisphere.

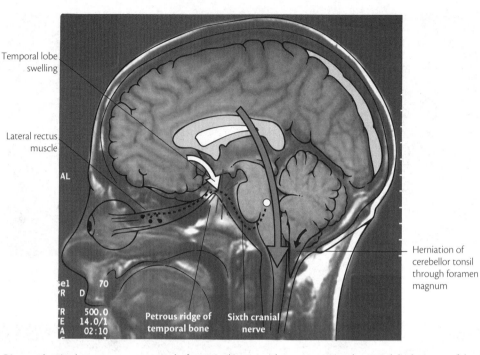

Fig. 7.10 Diagram showing how a pressure cone results from raised intracranial pressure, causing downward displacement of the swollen brain and plugging of the cerebellar tonsils in the foramen magnum. Also the sixth cranial nerve can become stretched, and compressed at the petrous ridge, causing loss of ocular abduction by the lateral rectus muscle.

Raised intracranial pressure

Sometimes raised intracranial pressure occurs because of the space-occupying effects of the tumour bulk, its surrounding oedema, and any secondary hydrocephalus. In adults the skull is an indistensible closed box and cannot expand to accommodate swollen contents. The skull can become grossly distended in infants who have developed brain swelling before natural fusion of their skull bone sutures. Generalized **headache** occurs which is worse in the morning or after lying down. Fundoscopy may show **papilloedema** of the optic nerve heads. High-dose steroid treatment with dexamethasone reduces the surrounding oedema.

Occasionally loss of ocular abduction due to a lateral rectus palsy develops as a **false localizing sign**. This occurs because the swollen brain compresses the sixth nerve as it crosses the petrous ridge of the temporal bone. Furthermore, the only direction the swollen brain can escape is downwards through the foramen magnum, which stretches the sixth nerve (Fig. 7.10).

Ultimately it is raised intracranial pressure which usually kills patients with brain tumours. Coma occurs because of diffuse damage to the brain. The cerebellar tonsils of the swollen brain expand downwards through the foramen magnum, a so-called '**pressure cone**', which compresses vital respiratory centres in the brainstem.

Treatment of brain tumours

Neurosurgery plays an important role in the diagnosis of most brain tumours, and sometimes in their treatment. Modern stereotactic biopsies are relatively non-traumatic. They provide a safe way of establishing the histological nature of the tumour and making sure it is not a cerebral abscess or a tuberculoma.

Radiotherapy rarely cures malignant glioma, but can extend survival modestly. Symptoms due to solitary cerebral metastases may be alleviated by neurosurgical removal and radiotherapy, but neurosurgery is not generally used for multiple cerebral secondary deposits from a known primary tumour. Meningiomas can be completely removed with permanent cure. Over 50 per cent of children with medulloblastoma survive 5 years after combination treatment by neurosurgical resection, radiotherapy, and chemotherapy.

CASE 7.1 'ANOTHER PROBLEM WITH STEROIDS'

A few weeks after visiting her family in Asia, a woman in her 60s developed unsteady gait, followed by headache and personality change. CT scan at a district general hospital revealed a ring-enhancing abnormality deep within the left frontal lobe. High-dose steroid therapy had been started before transfer to the neurosurgical department. Four days later, a stereotactic biopsy was undertaken by which time the enhancing mass was only half its original size (Fig. 7.11). The histology was inconclusive, showing no evi-dence of tumour, but a lymphoid infiltrate raised the question of tuberculoma. Anti-tuberculous therapy was started, along with phenytoin as prophylaxis against seizures. Eight days later the patient was referred to the neurology service with the question of phenytoin toxicity because of nausea, dizziness, and nystagmus. Dexamethasone was stopped for 16 days because of confusion about the underlying diagnosis. A further stereotactic biopsy showed a primary cere-bral lymphoma of B cell type.

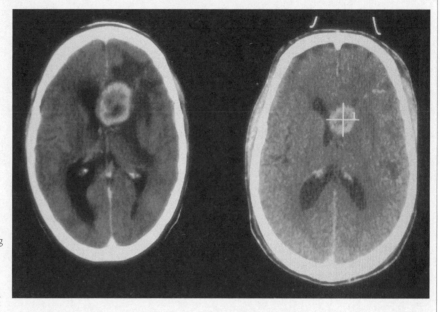

Fig. 7.11 Cerebral lymphoma. CT brain scan with contrast (left) before, and (right) 5 days after dexamethasone therapy. On steroids the frontal enhancing mass has shrunk markedly in size, with associated resolution of frontal oedema and unilateral hydrocephalus.

Comment

- Steroid therapy with dexamethasone reduces the oedema surrounding cerebral tumours. In so doing it can relieve the symptoms and signs of raised intracranial pressure.

- The size of a cerebral lymphoma is rapidly reduced by high-dose steroid therapy. But this can be at the expense of losing its distinctive histological appearance.

- The common practice in district general hospi-tals of starting steroids on first diagnosing a cerebral mass lesion can diminish the value of subsequent neurosurgical biopsy. It should be discouraged unless the patient needs treatment for significant symptoms of raised intracranial pressure due to cerebral oedema.

- Although cerebral lymphoma typically occurs in immunocompromised patients, such as transplant recipients or AIDS sufferers, it is increasingly common in the seemingly immuno-competent elderly.

- Despite an often dramatic early response of cerebral lymphoma to steroids and radiotherapy, the median survival is only 10–18 months even in immunocompetent patients.

CHAPTER 8

Weakness II: spinal cord lesions

Clinical features

The cardinal features of spinal cord disease are:

◆ bilateral leg weakness with extensor plantar responses;

◆ altered sphincter control;

◆ a sensory level (see Fig. 6.6, p. 48);

◆ weakness of the arms too if the lesion is high enough to affect the cervical spinal cord.

In well-established lesions, the tendon reflexes are brisk and ankle clonus is present, but these features do not develop until some days following an acute spinal cord lesion. In many spinal cord lesions the dorsal column sensory fibres will also be affected, causing abnormal joint position and vibration sensations in the feet with associated gait ataxia and a positive Romberg's test. Bladder control is lost as spinal cord disease becomes more severe. The sequence of events usually noticed by patients is, firstly, 'difficulty in walking' and later weakness, unsteadiness, and numbness or tingling of the feet, and ultimately becoming paraplegic with loss of sphincter control. Patients with suspected spinal cord compression must be investigated with MRI scanning promptly so as to avoid permanent spinal cord damage.

Causes of spinal cord lesions

There are four chief causes of a spinal cord lesion or 'myelopathy'.

1 **Spinal injuries** with spinal cord trauma due to fracture dislocation of the vertebral column (Fig. 8.1).

2 **Tumour** compressing the spinal cord. Extrinsic neural tumours such as **meningiomas** or **neurofibromas** can be removed completely by surgery (Fig. 8.13). Cord compression by secondary tumour

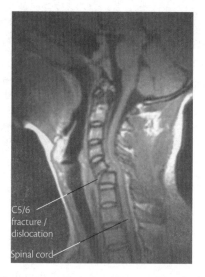

Fig. 8.1 Traumatic tetraplegia due to fracture–dislocation between the C5 and C6 vertebrae with spinal cord compression (MRI).

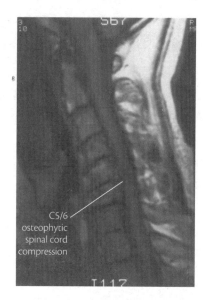

Fig. 8.3 Cervical spondylitic myelopathy showing spinal cord compression mainly by osteophytic outgrowths from the vertebral bodies at the C5/C6 level, and to a lesser extent at the C4/C5 level (MRI).

deposits in vertebral bones (Fig. 8.2), usually derived from prostatic or breast carcinoma or myeloma, are better treated by radiotherapy and chemotherapy than by surgical decompression; however, permanent cure rarely results.

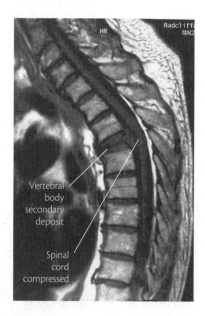

Fig. 8.2 A T7 vertebral body carcinoma deposit, with vertebral collapse and compression of the spinal cord (MRI).

3 **Cervical spondylitic myelopathy.** Combinations of intervertebral disc prolapse, osteophytic bone protrusions, and spondylolisthetic slippage between vertebrae is a common cause of slowly progressive cervical myelopathy. It usually affects patients over 50. Single or multiple levels of the spinal cord may be compressed between the third and seventh cervical vertebrae (Fig. 8.3). Often the spondylosis also compresses nerve roots to the arms, in which case the entire clinical picture is described as a 'cervical spondylitic radiculo-myelopathy'.

4 **Myelitis** is a medical disease due to intrinsic demyelination and/or inflammation of the spinal cord. It is usually seen as part of multiple sclerosis, in which it often causes the principal disability. But myelitis can occur as an isolated phenomenon which usually recovers spontaneously, although sometimes incompletely.

Diagnosis

Establishing the level of the lesion

It is important to identify the level of a spinal cord lesion for possible neurosurgical treatment. Much can be achieved on simple clinical grounds. It is crucial to establish the **sensory level**, which is best done by moving up the legs and trunk with a pin and asking the patient 'tell me when you feel this pin as properly sharp'. Most spinal cord compression due to tumour

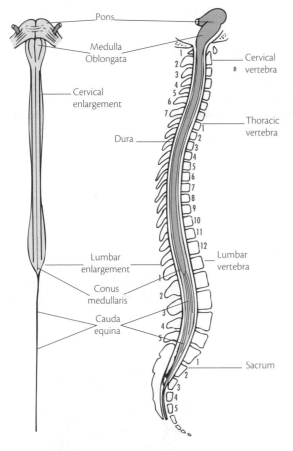

Fig. 8.4 Diagram showing how the spinal cord is shorter than the spinal canal, and ends at the L1 or sometimes L2 vertebral body. This means that lumbar puncture to obtain CSF samples can be undertaken safely at the L3/L4 level and below.

affects the thoracic spine and you should remember the following landmark dermatomes (groin skin crease T12–L1, umbilicus T10, costal margin T6, nipple T4, armpit T2). When ascribing these neurological levels to a corresponding vertebral abnormality, one should remember that the spinal cord is much shorter than the spinal canal and indeed ends at the level of the L1 vertebra (Fig. 8.4). Thus, in the thoracic region, the vertebral level corresponding to a lesion is about two segments above the dermatomal sensory level mapped on the skin.

Spinal cord imaging

Although plain spine X-rays may reveal spondylosis or vertebral bone abnormalities potentially compressing the spinal cord, proof of spinal cord compression requires imaging by myelography or MRI. Myelography involved injection by lumbar puncture of radio-opaque contrast medium into the spinal fluid, which then outlined the spinal cord and roots (Fig. 11.4). It has been replaced by non-invasive MRI, which clearly demarcates all causes of spinal cord compression, and can also show plaques of demyelination within the spinal cord in myelitis.

Unusual patterns of sensory loss due to spinal cord lesions

When interpreting the sensory loss due to partial spinal cord lesions, it is important to remember that **joint position** and **vibration sensations** are carried ipsilaterally in the dorsal columns whereas **temperature** and **pain sensations** are carried contralaterally within the spinothalamic tract (Fig. 8.5).

Syringomyelia

In syringomyelia, a fluid-filled cavity within the central spinal cord disrupts the decussating spinothalamic

Fig. 8.5 Cross-section of spinal cord showing the position of the descending pyramidal tract, containing upper motor neuron axons. The ascending sensory pathways of the dorsal column (uncrossed), which decussate after synapsing in the gracile and cuneate nuclei, and the spinothalamic tract (crossed) are also shown.

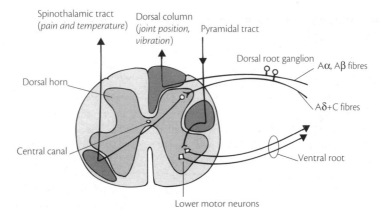

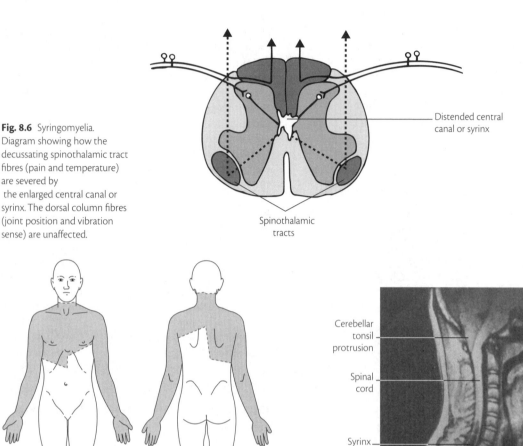

Fig. 8.6 Syringomyelia. Diagram showing how the decussating spinothalamic tract fibres (pain and temperature) are severed by the enlarged central canal or syrinx. The dorsal column fibres (joint position and vibration sense) are unaffected.

Distended central canal or syrinx

Spinothalamic tracts

Fig. 8.7 A 'cape-like' pattern of suspended pain and temperature loss in syringomyelia affecting the cervical and upper thoracic segments of the spinal cord.

Cerebellar tonsil protrusion

Spinal cord

Syrinx cavity

Fig. 8.8 A syringomyelia cavity in the lower cervical spinal cord associated with a Chiari malformation, a congenital anomaly in which the cerebellar tonsils protrude through the foramen magnum (MRI).

tract fibres (Fig. 8.6). This causes **dissociated sensory loss** with loss of pain and temperature sensations, but preserved joint position and vibration senses carried by the dorsal columns (Fig. 8.7).

Syringomyelia most usually affects the lower cervical and upper thoracic spinal cord. It initially causes loss of pain and temperature sensation on the hands and allows painless burns to occur. Later the syrinx may extend to disrupt tendon reflex arcs and cause motor neuron degeneration, leading to wasting of the small hand muscles. It may be associated with a congenital anomaly of the cerebellum, a Chiari malformation, in which the cerebellar tonsils protrude through the foramen magnum (Fig. 8.8).

Brown–Séquard syndrome

A Brown–Séquard syndrome follows damage to one half of the spinal cord (Fig. 8.9). Below the level of the damage, this produces ipsilateral weakness and loss of vibration and joint position sensations, with contralateral loss of temperature and pain sensations. Brown–Séquard syndromes are usually due to trauma, ischaemia, focal myelitis or radiation damage.

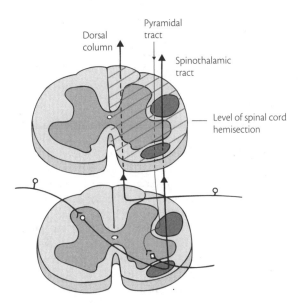

Fig. 8.9 A Brown–Séquard syndrome due to hemisection of the spinal cord. There is ipsilateral weakness due to pyramidal tract damage, ipsilateral loss of joint position and vibration sensations due to dorsal column damage, and contralateral loss of pain and temperature sensation due to spinothalamic tract damage.

Anterior spinal artery occlusion

Anterior spinal artery occlusion usually affects the mid or lower thoracic spinal cord due to occlusion of the artery of Adamkewitz, its main feeding branch from the abdominal aorta. Such occlusions often complicate abdominal aortic aneurism surgery, or occur spontaneously in atherosclerosis. Because the arterial territory involves only the front half of the spinal cord, the pyramidal and spinothalamic tracts are damaged, but

the dorsal columns are not (Fig. 8.10). This causes bilateral weakness with loss of pain and temperature appreciation below the lesion, whereas vibration and joint position sensations are preserved. Associated infarction of the anterior horns of the spinal cord at the level of the lesion also produces a lower motor neuron lesion affecting the muscles locally at that level.

Sphincter disturbance

Rapidly evolving spinal cord lesions cause hesitancy of micturition and finally retention of urine and faeces. Chronic spinal cord lesions cause symptoms of urgency, or involuntary reflex voiding, yet bladder emptying is usually incomplete with large residual volumes of urine. These difficulties may be compounded by associated immobility which prevents speedy visits to the lavatory.

Damage to the nerve roots of the cauda equina causes a flaccid bladder with loss of urethral and bladder sensation, numbness of the perineum, and a flaccid insensitive anus.

Bladders with large residual volumes of stagnant urine are prone to infection. This can lead to chronic renal failure when coupled with back pressure and ureteric reflux. To overcome this, patients can be taught intermittent self-catheterization, or chronically indwelling urinary catheters may be inserted, often suprapubically.

Sexual impotence results from both spinal cord and cauda equina lesions.

Satisfactory automatic bowel actions can be established by judicious diet, by bulking agents and softeners, and by promoting reflex evacuation by warm drinks such as tea. However, patients frequently have to resort to manual evacuation of faeces.

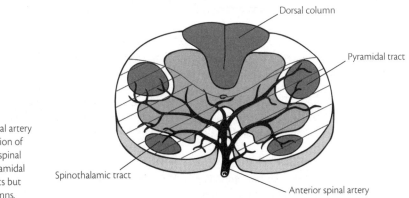

Fig. 8.10 Anterior spinal artery occlusion causes infarction of the anterior half of the spinal cord, damaging the pyramidal and spinothalamic tracts but sparing the dorsal columns.

Multiple sclerosis

Multiple Sclerosis causes a **relapsing and remitting** pattern of attacks of neurological disturbance affecting different parts of the central nervous system at different points in time. Multiple sclerosis is a major cause of disability amongst those of working age. It has a prevalence of 1:1000 in the UK population. The neurological dysfunction is due to plaques of **demyelination** in the central nervous system white matter. These are particularly common in the optic nerves, cervical spinal cord, periventricular cerebral white matter, and the brainstem. This demyelination blocks conduction of impulses along the axons within the affected plaque with resultant loss of function.

After the phase of acute demyelination, which generally deteriorates over 12 hours to 5 days, there is a plateau of stable disability for roughly 1–4 weeks before a degree of remyelination occurs with partial recovery of symptoms over the next few weeks or months. Recovery by remyelination from an individual attack is rarely complete, although fortunately it is often considerable. Severe attacks can cause considerable axonal damage in addition to demyelination. Thus, with frequent or severe relapses, permanent background disability accumulates.

Causation

The precise cause of multiple sclerosis remains unknown. It is generally believed to be either immunologically or virally mediated, possibly an interaction of both. **Genetic factors** thought to involve immune response genes lead to relative risks for identical twins of 1 in 3, and siblings of 1 in 20. Overall, 1 in 50 patients has an affected first-degree relative. Discussion of these family risks is increasingly requested by patients and their relatives. Females are more commonly affected than men. Only rarely does the disease start before puberty or after middle age. An ill-understood **environmental factor** seems to play a part too. The incidence increases with geographical latitude such that it is rare in the tropics and common in temperate regions. If you migrate from one to the other before your mid-teens, you tend to acquire the risk of the region to which you have moved. Migration after the mid-teens means that you carry your pre-existing risk. The disease was unknown in the Faroe Islands before troops were stationed there in the Second World War, which suggests an infective component.

Clinical picture

A huge variety of neurological disturbances can occur in multiple sclerosis and no two patients run the same clinical course. The commonest manifestations are optic neuritis, spinal cord lesions, brainstem demyelination, and eye movement abnormalities. Dysphasia, hemiplegia, deafness, and extrapyramidal movement disorders are all unusual.

Optic neuritis

Optic neuritis is also known as **retrobulbar neuritis**, or **acute papillitis**. Unilateral optic nerve demyelination causes loss of visual acuity. Loss or degeneration of colour vision is prominent. Various visual field defects occur, the most usual of which is a central scotoma. There may be retro-ocular pain on eye movement. If the demyelinating plaque is situated at the junction with the eyeball, fundoscopy may show a swollen optic nerve head, an appearance known as **papillitis**. Papillitis and papilloedema look similar, but visual acuity is well preserved in papilloedema, which is usually bilateral. Optic neuritis can occur as an isolated phenomenon in many patients who never go on to develop multiple sclerosis.

Spinal cord lesions (or myelitis)

These cause limb weakness which varies in severity from acute tetraplegia or paraplegia to a mild monoparesis affecting one limb. More commonly, myelitis simply produces a patch of numbness or tingling on a limb which may spread onto the adjacent trunk over the next few days (see Fig. 6.5, p. 47). Myelitis affecting the dorsal columns can produce a disabling sensory ataxia of one hand or of the legs. Sphincter control can be affected, and urinary urgency or retention, or altered sexual function, can be the sole manifestations of an attack. These differing manifestations of myelitis depend on the plaque's size, its location, and which pathways it affects within the spinal cord.

Brainstem demyelination

Demyelination of brainstem, cerebellar and vestibular pathways causes vertigo or ataxia. Sometimes the arm ataxia can be particularly wild and disabling.

Eye movement abnormalities

Eye movement abnormalities due to brainstem demyelination are usually of three types: **jerk nystagmus** on lateral gaze; **gaze palsies** in which the eyes cannot make a yoked gaze movement to look in a particular direction; and **internuclear ophthalmoplegia** in which one eye cannot adduct during a lateral gaze movement normally involving both eyes.

Diagnosis

Making the diagnosis of clinically definite multiple sclerosis requires clear evidence of at least two definite attacks at different times, affecting different parts of the nervous system. Some patients may only have two minor attacks in their entire life. Others may develop a very fulminant form and become severely disabled by multiple attacks during the first year. Most patients fall between these two extremes. Many patients eventually develop slowly **progressive spinal cord damage** some years after the relapsing/remitting phase of the disorder. This secondary progressive spinal cord disease is the most common cause of serious disability.

Sometimes demyelination is suggested by worsening of symptoms during hot baths or exercise, so-called **Uhtoff's phenomenon**.

Lhermitte's symptom consists of shooting electric shock sensations or tinglings down the limbs provoked by flexing the neck. Although this strongly suggests multiple sclerosis it can occur in other conditions affecting the cervical spinal cord, including cervical spondylosis and subacute combined demyelination of the spinal cord due to vitamin B$_{12}$ deficiency.

Although MRI and autopsy studies frequently show extensive plaques throughout the cerebral hemispheres, major cognitive and psychiatric abnormalities are relatively uncommon in multiple sclerosis. Only occasionally does multiple sclerosis cause marked dementia. Sometimes rather disabled patients seem relatively unconcerned by their plight; maybe this is due to lack of insight as a result of frontal lobe demyelination.

Someone who has only ever had one attack of demyelination does not have multiple sclerosis, although they may later develop it. Thus critical clinical assessment is vital for making the diagnosis. The following two investigations can provide support for the clinical diagnosis.

MRI of the brain

MRI of the brain may show typical periventricular demyelination (Fig. 8.11). If this MRI appearance is seen in a patient who has had a first and only attack of either optic neuritis, brainstem disease, or a spinal cord lesion, there is approximately a 60 per cent chance of clinically definite multiple sclerosis developing within 5 years. On the other hand, if periventricular demyelination is absent in such patients, their risk of multiple sclerosis is only about 10 per cent at 5 years.

Visual evoked potentials

Visual evoked potentials measure the speed of impulse conduction along the optic nerves to the visual cortex in response to an alternating chequerboard pattern. Slowing due to demyelination may remain for many

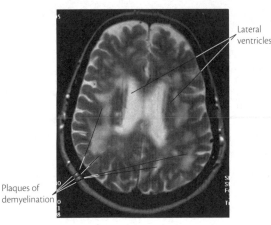

Fig. 8.11 Cerebral hemisphere plaques of demyelination in multiple sclerosis (MRI).

years, or forever, after a single attack of optic neuritis (Fig. 8.12). Sometimes an attack of optic neuritis has been asymptomatic. In such cases, visual evoked potentials provide useful adjunctive evidence for multiple sclerosis by demonstrating the presence of a second lesion.

Cerebrospinal fluid (CSF)

During clinically active phases of the disease, increased CSF protein and lymphocyte counts, rarely exceeding 50 cells/mm^3 (normal <5/mm^3) are common. CSF electrophoresis reveals an **oligoclonal banding pattern** in most patients with multiple sclerosis. This can be

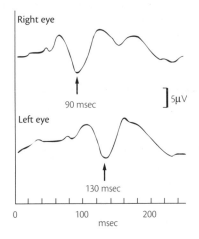

Fig. 8.12 Visual evoked potential (VEP) showing a prolonged latency on the left of about 130 milliseconds in a patient with left optic neuritis.

diagnostically helpful in older patients when faced with the differential diagnosis of cerebrovascular disease or cervical spondylitic myelopathy.

Managing a patient with multiple sclerosis

Nowadays most patients expect the diagnosis to be named and for a frank discussion of what the future holds, how it may affect life expectancy, what are the risks to relatives, and whether it is safe to become pregnant. Because prognostication in multiple sclerosis is notoriously unreliable, many questions can be answered only in general terms. Many patients presume that multiple sclerosis inevitably causes severe disability. They should be reassured that some patients go through life with only a handful of attacks, and never develop a serious lasting disability. Unsurprisingly, life expectancy is reduced in those with severe disability who develop severe complications such as sphincter disorders or infected pressure sores. Multiple sclerosis is not a contraindication to **pregnancy**, although this may pose practical difficulties for a mother if significantly disabled. Although the risk of a relapse is reduced during the pregnancy itself, the risks during the puerperium are increased, making the overall risk roughly the same as normal.

Disabling acute relapses may be treated with intravenous or oral steroids. This speeds recovery, but probably does not improve the eventual extent of recovery.

Prophylactic treatment

Clinical trials have examined a wide range of immunosuppressant therapies without identifying any which clearly retard the accumulation of disability in multiple sclerosis. Beta interferon has recently been identified as an injectable drug which can reduce the relapse rate by roughly one-third, but it is not certain whether it has a beneficial effect in preventing disability.

Managing paraplegia

This involves principles applicable to chronic spinal cord lesions of all causes.

1 **Mobility** is most effectively preserved by wheelchairs once walking has been lost.

2 **Spasticity** can be reduced by drugs such as baclofen or diazepam. However, one must guard against making the legs weak and jelly-like, thereby making them even less useful for walking. Severe spasticity of the thigh adductor muscles can impede toileting and be relieved by local botulinum toxin injections.

3 **Feeding**: thick handle grips on cutlery can enable quadriparetic patients to feed independently.

4 **Cerebellar tremor** in multiple sclerosis is extremely difficult to treat effectively. It is particularly disabling when combined with quadriparesis. It can cause severe disability and even self-injury.

5 **Spincter disturbances**: the treatment of bladder and bowel dysfunction has been outlined above.

6 **Bed sores** should be avoided by providing suitably padded wheelchairs, and turning immobile patients every few hours to avoid prolonged pressure on hip or ischial bones.

7 A **care team**, led by a consultant in neurological disability, may provide appliances to overcome specific disabilities and modify the home so that patients can remain living at home despite severe disability. This often puts a considerable burden on the spouse or carer. Particular modifications with a practical value include the provision of handrails for patients to permit walking inside the house, hoists and other modifications for the bathroom, and wheelchair access ramps.

CASE 8.1 'FIRST ONE LIMB, THEN THE OTHERS'

For 2 years a 45-year-old woman developed progressive deadness and tingling of the fingertips on her right hand, with loss of manipulatory ability and weakness of grip. For the past few months she had had intermittent tinglings in the right leg and the left hand too. Examination showed only an absent right plantar response and slightly reduced pinprick sensation in the right hand and foot. This syndrome of progressive 'rotating sensory loss' starting in one limb and spreading to those adjacent, suggested a compressive lesion of the upper cervical cord around the foramen magnum. MRI (Fig. 8.13) showed an intraspinal, extra-axial solid tumour at the level of the first and second cervical vertebrae, causing considerable spinal cord compression. This neurofibroma was removed neurosurgically. Her limb symptoms recovered well, although she was left with unilateral numbness on the back of the head because the neurofibroma had arisen from a C2 nerve root.

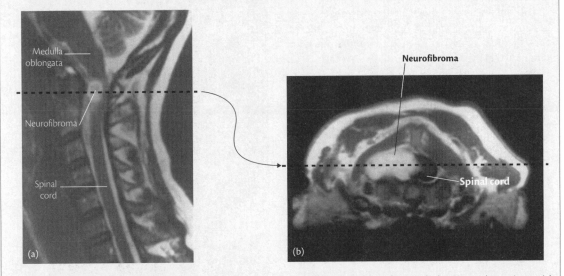

Fig. 8.13 A neurofibroma compressing the cervical spinal cord at the C2 level. (a) Sagittal MRI showing the location at the cervicocranial junction. (b) Transverse MRI showing the origin of the tumour from a C2 nerve root to one side of the spinal canal.

Comment

- Sensory loss rotating progressively from limb to limb is strongly suggestive of a compressive lesion of the upper cervical spinal cord. It can also occur with myelitis due to demyelination.

- Anatomically severe spinal cord compression and deviation, as shown by this MRI, can be associated with a relative paucity of physical signs. This is particularly likely if it develops slowly.

- Good recovery ensues if the spinal cord is decompressed before signs of long tract damage have emerged. In contrast once a patient has developed significant limb weakness, or disturbed control of micturition, one must be guarded about the extent to which functional recovery will follow anatomically satisfactory decompression.

CASE 8.2 'THE WINNING TRY'

A 30-year-old rugby forward peeled off a loose maul, and dived full length to score a try with his outstretched right hand. In so doing he banged his head into an opposing forward's knee. As his jubilant team mates returned to the half-way line, and the dejected opposition retired to await the conversion attempt, our hero remained outstretched in his scoring position. He had total paralysis and loss of sensation from the neck down. Within 1 hour limb movements returned and within 3 days he was able to walk with a frame but still required a urinary catheter. He had the typical signs of a cervical spinal cord lesion with moderate tetraparesis, extensor plantar responses, and absent abdominal reflexes. Sensation had largely returned but pinprick remained diminished in the right leg. Whereas most of the tendon reflexes were brisk, the biceps (C5–C6) reflexes were absent, suggesting local damage to the reflex arc in the spinal cord at the C5/C6 level. Fortunately, plain X-ray of the cervical spine did not reveal vertebral fracture–dislocation. MRI showed a generally narrow cervical spinal canal, without significant intervertebral disc prolapse, and without compression of the spinal cord. However, there was a small patch of oedema in the spinal cord opposite the C3/C4 disc space (Fig. 8.14). In view of this it was hypothesized that a momentary central protrusion of the C3/C4 disc had occurred when he had banged his head during scoring and this had traumatized the spinal cord. He went on to recover nearly completely, marred only by some residual tingling sensations and cold sensitivity of his limbs, and minor weakness of his left arm.

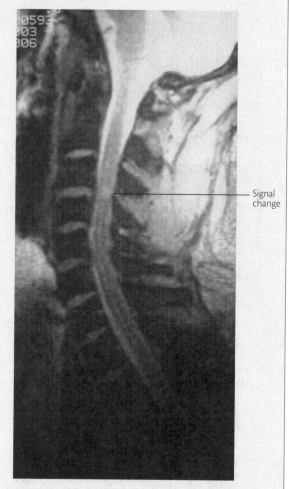

Signal change

Fig. 8.14 MRI of the cervical spine showing a patch of signal change in the mid-cervical spinal cord. This was attributed to trauma caused by temporary protrusion of the adjacent C3/C4 intervertebral disc at the time of head and neck trauma.

Comment

♦ This man was very lucky. Most traumatic damage to the cervical spinal cord occurs with fracture–dislocations of the vertebrae which do not resolve spontaneously. This leaves substantial or complete weakness with a life of chronic disability.

♦ Along with motor cycle and other road traffic accidents, the leading causes of traumatic spinal cord injury are sporting injuries often in rugby or when diving into shallow water.

♦ This man's instantaneous onset of spinal paralysis could only be explained by momentary spinal cord compression. Other causes of instantaneous neurological deficits, such as epilepsy or ruptured arteries, were not possible explanations here.

Weakness III: nerve root lesions

Sensorimotor symptoms in one limb

It is common for patients to complain of pain, altered sensation, weakness, or difficulty in using a limb. First you need to be sure that these aren't due to joint or tendon disease. That would be suggested by local tenderness, restricted passive joint movements, and clear localization of pain to a moving joint or tendon. Having excluded joint disease, you need to distinguish between nerve root, focal peripheral nerve, and plexus lesions as causes for such symptoms.

Nerve root lesions

Nerve root lesions are usually due to **prolapsed intervertebral disc**. The predominant sensory symptom is a **shooting pain** within the distribution of a particular root: to the point of the shoulder (C5 root), to the thumb and index finger (C6), to the middle finger (C7), sciatica down the lateral thigh and calf and dorsum of foot (L5), sciatica down the posterolateral thigh and posterior calf (S1). Coughing, sneezing, or straining often exacerbates the radicular pain in prolapsed intervertebral disc.

1 Focal **muscle wasting** may be noted in established root lesions, but weakness is not usually a prominent early symptom.

2 **Areflexia** will correspond to the root affected by the lesion.

3 Frequently there is **spine pain** which corresponds to the level of a slipped intervertebral disc or spondylitic root compression.

4 **Straight leg raising** is restricted to less than the normal 90° by pain in lumbosacral root compression by slipped disc.

Focal peripheral nerve lesions

Ulnar and **median nerve** compression in the arm usually cause paraesthesia rather than the shooting pain of

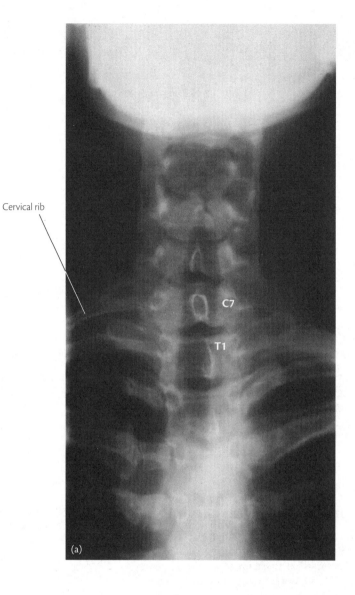

Cervical rib

C7

T1

(a)

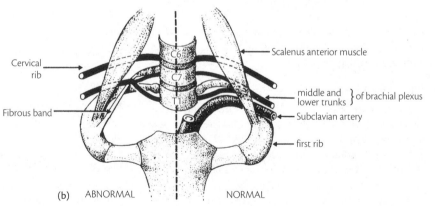

Fig. 9.1 Thoracic outlet syndrome due to cervical rib. (a) Plain X-ray of the cervical spine showing a rib emanating from the C7 transverse process. Note that the C7 transverse process is downturned whereas the transverse process of T1 is upturned. (b) Diagram showing (left) how the lower brachial plexus can be distorted by cervical rib or associated fibrous band. However, most cervical ribs remain asymptomatic throughout life.

Cervical rib

Fibrous band

(b)   ABNORMAL

C6

C7

T1

Scalenus anterior muscle

middle and } of brachial plexus
lower trunks }

Subclavian artery

first rib

NORMAL

a root lesion. These paraesthesiae may be uncomfortable. Although muscle wasting occurs, affecting the dorsal interosseous muscles (ulnar nerve) or thenar eminence (median), it often goes unnoticed by the patient. **Common peroneal nerve** lesions usually present with painless flaccid footdrop. The reflexes remain normal because these peripheral nerve lesions are too distal to involve the reflex arc. Nerve conduction studies show focal conduction block at the site of the lesion: in the cubital canal at the elbow (ulnar nerve), in the carpal tunnel at the wrist (median), or at the fibular head (common peroneal).

Brachial and lumbosacral plexus lesions

In general, you should suspect a plexus lesion when combinations of motor, sensory, and reflex loss do not correspond to the territory of an individual peripheral nerve or root. The brachial plexus is prone to stretch injury by shoulder avulsion during breech delivery, or in motorcycle accidents. In contrast, the lumbosacral plexus is protected from trauma by the bony pelvic ring. Metastatic tumour deposits can infiltrate either plexus causing severe pain. Painless progressive weakness may occur years after radiotherapy fields have included a plexus.

The brachial plexus can be compressed from below by a cervical rib articulating with the C7 vertebral body (Fig. 9.1). The resultant **thoracic outlet syndrome** involves pain and sensory loss on the ulnar side of the hand (fifth finger) coupled with wasting and weakness of the thenar eminence. In other words a pattern that cannot be explained by an individual peripheral nerve, or nerve root, lesion.

Prolapsed (or slipped) intervertebral disc

This is due to rupture of the nucleus pulposus through the annulus fibrosis of an intervertebral disc. If the rupture occurs into the central spinal canal (Fig. 9.2(b); **central disc prolapse**) it will compress the spinal cord in the cervical region or the cauda equina in the lumbar canals. A lateral rupture affects the nerve roots entering and leaving the intervertebral foramen (Fig. 9.2(c); **lateral disc prolapse**).

Lateral disc prolapse most commonly affects the L5/S1 disc (compressing the S1 root) or the L4/L5 disc (L5 root) in the lumbosacral spine. Less frequently the C5/C6 (C6 root) or C6/C7 (C7 root) discs are affected in the neck. Disc prolapse may be precipitated by activity or trauma. It is associated with local articular pain and limitation of movement in the spine. When disc prolapse compresses nerve roots it produces severe radiating pain down the back of the leg, which is known as **sciatica**, or similar pain across the shoulder and down the arm. This combination of severe radiating radicular pain and spinal ache frequently prostrates patients.

Slipped disc can be proved by MRI. This shows the prolapsed disc obliterating or narrowing the intervertebral foramen (Fig. 9.3).

Treatment

Treatment of slipped disc may be either conservative or surgical. The conservative approach uses analgesics and immobilization of the affected spinal segment with a surgical collar for the neck, or by prolonged bed rest for the lumbar spine. Conservative treatment is often suc-

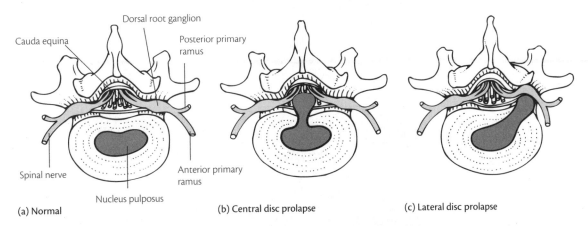

(a) Normal
(b) Central disc prolapse
(c) Lateral disc prolapse

Cauda equina
Dorsal root ganglion
Posterior primary ramus
Spinal nerve
Nucleus pulposus
Anterior primary ramus

Fig. 9.2 (b) Central and (c) lateral prolapse of a lumbar intervertebral disc causing compression of (b) the cauda equina and (c) the exiting nerve root, respectively.

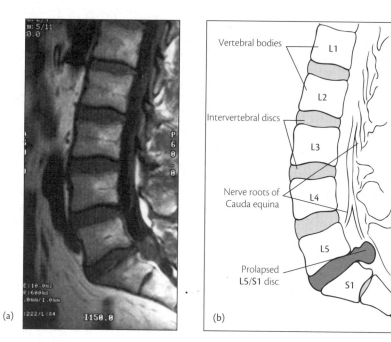

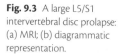

Fig. 9.3 A large L5/S1 intervertebral disc prolapse: (a) MRI; (b) diagrammatic representation.

(a)

(b)

cessful, but the patient remains at risk of recurrent episodes with considerable loss of time from work and recreation. Neurosurgical disc removal provides more definitive treatment of the pain, and increasingly it is offered in a first episode. Neither conservative nor surgical treatment will restore much muscle power when motor root involvement has caused weakness. Thus, even after pain has been successfully treated, a foot-

drop (L5 root) may remain and cause patients to catch their toe whilst walking; or plantar reflexion weakness (S1 root) may take the spring out of their stride; or weak elbow extension (C7 root) may make it difficult to find third gear whilst driving, or weak elbow flexion (C6) may make it difficult to lift things.

Central disc prolapse into the lumbar canal can cause acute cauda equina compression with altered

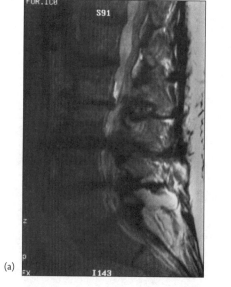

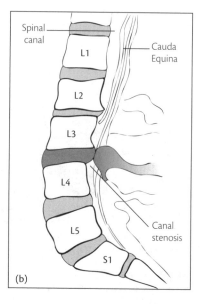

Fig. 9.4 Lumbar canal stenosis compressing the cauda equina at L3/L4 due to osteophytes, ligament hypertrophy, and disc prolapse. (a) MRI; (b) diagrammatic representation.

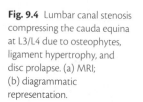

(a)

(b)

bladder control, weak legs, and diminished sacral sensation. This is an emergency requiring immediate MRI with a view to urgent neurosurgical decompression.

Lumbar canal stenosis

This causes a disabling walking disorder in the elderly. It is quite common and is treatable by a relatively straightforward and well-tolerated operation. The condition causes numbness, discomfort, and weakness of the legs which develop whilst walking or during prolonged standing. Yet these symptoms do not develop during similar exercise with the back flexed during cycling. These patients are suffering from intermittent cauda equina compression due to stenosis of the lumbar spinal canal which is maximized by the erect posture. The stenosis is due to combinations of slipped intervertebral disc, spondylolisthesis (slippage between adjacent vertebrae), hypertrophy of the intraspinal ligaments, and spondylitic protrusions from vertebral bones, often superimposed on a canal which was congenitally rather narrow (Fig. 9.4). Spinal canal stenosis can be diagnosed reliably by MRI.

Patients with spinal stenosis sometimes complain of sciatica or impaired bladder control too. You may be able to demonstrate that abnormal neurological signs appear after walking, such as absent ankle jerks or weakness of ankle dorsiflexion. The patient's walking distance decreases as the stenosis worsens over months and years. Patients stop walking and sit down for a few minutes to relieve symptoms. Surgical laminectomy to remove the back of the narrowed portion of the spinal canal improves symptoms in many patients. Spinal canal stenosis is an important cause of reversible disability in the elderly.

The symptoms of spinal canal stenosis must be distinguished from those of **vascular intermittent claudication** due to atheromatous narrowing of the ilio-femoral–popliteal arteries. This usually involves a deep-seated aching pain in the calves on exercise which is relieved by simply standing still rather than by sitting down. Vascular intermittent claudication is usually associated with absent dorsalis pedis pulses, and poor perfusion of the foot skin.

CASE 9.1 'AN INCOMPLETE CLINICAL PICTURE'

A normally athletic teenage boy had lost his previous sprinting speed over 2 years. In recent months his walking also slowed, and he started scuffing his toes and tripping due to slight foot drop on the left. There were no sensory symptoms, all his sphincter functions were normal, and his hands were unaffected. Examination showed weakness and slight wasting of all the leg muscles below the knees with an absent left ankle jerk and flexor plantar responses. There was a hint of reduced temperature sensation on the dorsum of the left foot. Although he had been referred with nerve conduction studies interpreted as showing a pure motor polyneuropathy, such disorders usually predominate in the arms, which were completely normal. MRI of the lumbar spinal canal showed an intradural extramedullary mass opposite the L1 vertebra posterior to the conus medullaris (Fig. 9.5). Neurosurgical removal of this neurofibroma allowed substantial recovery of leg function, and he became able to play football again, although with some residual ankle dorsal flexion weakness on the left.

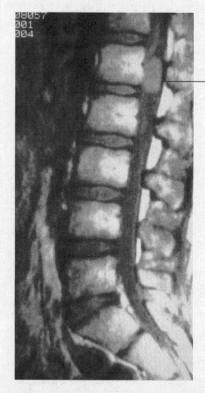

Fig. 9.5 MRI showing a neurofibroma at the level of the L1 vertebra compressing the conus medullaris and upper cauda equina.

Conus neurofibroma

Comment

- If a patient's clinical features are not consistent with the putative diagnosis, take the history again from scratch, examine the patient carefully and with an open mind, and investigate other possible diagnoses.

- This boy's weakness was restricted to the legs, and the clinical and electrophysiological features had not supported the diagnosis of generalized peripheral neuropathy. Furthermore, the asymmetrical leg muscle involvement and the minor sensory disturbance were not typical of a spinal muscular atrophy, which is an inherited or acquired degeneration of lower motor neurons.

- One expects compressive tumours of the cauda equina nerve roots to produce leg sensory disturbance and abnormal sphincter control in addition to muscle weakness; that is the full-blown syndrome. Compression higher in the spinal canal at the level of the conus medullaris of the spinal cord would be expected to produce extensor plantars. The lesson is that such compression syndromes may be clinically incomplete, particularly in the early stages.

- Increasingly nowadays, patients seek medical advice before they have progressed to the 'full-house' of symptoms and signs diagnostic of a particular disorder. Modern neurology needs to investigate the possible diseases which could be the cause of such incomplete, early syndromes. For, in cases like this, it is early decompression that will allow good recovery and forestall permanent severe disability.

CHAPTER 10

Weakness IV: focal peripheral nerve lesions

Types of peripheral neuropathy

Lesions of peripheral nerves cause varying combinations of sensory loss, muscle weakness, reflex loss, and autonomic loss, depending upon which axon type is mainly affected and at what point along its length. You should distinguish two main anatomical distributions of peripheral neuropathy:

1 **Focal neuropathy** affects the nerve fibres of the trunk of an individual peripheral nerve.

2 **Polyneuropathy** affects all nerve fibres equally, irrespective of which peripheral nerve they are in, producing a generalized and symmetrical abnormality

Focal neuropathy or mononeuropathy

Focal neuropathy reflects a lesion of an individual peripheral nerve, such as the median nerve. It usually occurs due to **trauma** which may sever the nerve; due to **compression** by a tendon as in the carpal tunnel syndrome; or due to **external pressure** as in a Saturday night palsy wrist drop from compression of the radial nerve against the humerus as the arm is sprawled across the arm of a chair whilst in a drunken stupor.

Less frequently, mononeuropathy results from focal blockage of small blood vessels supplying a nerve, the 'vasa nervorum', causing ischaemic damage. This usually results from **diabetes mellitus** or from inflammatory **vasculitis**; measurement of the blood sugar and erythrocyte sedimentation rate are advisable in all focal neuropathies. In both these conditions a number of different nerves may be affected causing '**mononeuritis multiplex**'.

If focal peripheral neuropathy merely involves localized demyelination, full recovery occurs 6–10 weeks after relieving the pressure, a so-called '**neurapraxia**'.

However, if axons have been severed by trauma, severe compression or infarction, recovery can only occur by axonal regeneration. This proceeds at 1 mm/day at best, and is often incomplete.

The common focal peripheral nerve lesions that are encountered are:

1 **Median** at the wrist causing carpal tunnel syndrome with a painful tingly hand at night. Weakness of abductor pollicis brevis and sensory diminution over the tips of the thumb, index and middle fingers may be demonstrable.

2 **Ulnar** in the cubital canal at the elbow causing sensory loss on the little finger and half of the ring finger, and weakness of dorsal interosseous muscles.

3 **Radial** above the elbow causing weakness of finger and wrist extension and a small patch of sensory loss on the dorsum of the thumb.

4 **Common peroneal** at the fibular head causing foot drop and sensory loss over the dorsum of the foot and lateral shin.

5 **Lateral cutaneous nerve of the thigh** at the inguinal ligament with sensory loss over the anterolateral thigh, which may become painful on walking, known as 'meralgia paraesthetica'.

The skin territories supplied by these nerves are shown in Fig. 6.2 (p. 47).

Carpal tunnel syndrome

This common mononeuropathy is due to compression of the median nerve as it passes under the transverse carpal ligament at the wrist. It usually affects middle-aged women. Typically they complain of painful tingling in the thumb and first three fingers which awakens them at night or is provoked by manual tasks such as writing or sewing. Many patients are unable to identify accurately which fingers are affected. Often no physical signs are demonstrable. You should look for weakness and wasting of abductor policis brevis (median nerve) (Fig. 10.1), whereas dorsal interosseous muscle power (ulnar nerve) should be normal. Pinprick sensory loss may be present in the median three and a half digits (Fig. 10.2).

Carpal tunnel syndrome may be symptomatic of hypothyroidism, acromegaly, Cushing's disease, rheumatoid arthritis, pregnancy, or repetitive use of vibrating tools. The diagnosis is proved by nerve conduction studies. Motor conduction velocity is slowed in the median nerve through the carpal tunnel despite the forearm conduction of velocity being normal (see Fig. 11.3, p. 83). The symptoms are usually abolished by surgical release of the transverse carpal ligament under local anaesthesia. Less severe symptoms can be relieved by steroid injection into the carpal tunnel.

Ulnar nerve lesions

These usually occur at the elbow as the nerve passes through the cubital canal distal to the medial epicondyle groove. Often the cause is a tight tendinous roof to the canal, or external pressure upon a nerve which dislocates out of the groove when leaning on bent elbows. Patients complain of tingling and deadness in the little and ring fingers, and the ulnar border of the hand (Fig. 10.3).

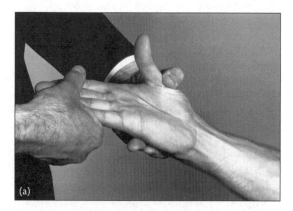

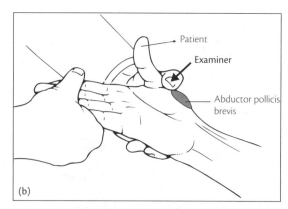

Fig. 10.1 Testing the power of abductor pollicis brevis (median nerve) and observing its bulk. The patient should raise their thumb at right angles from their palm, and the examiner should oppose this movement by pressing down at the base of the proximal phalanx.

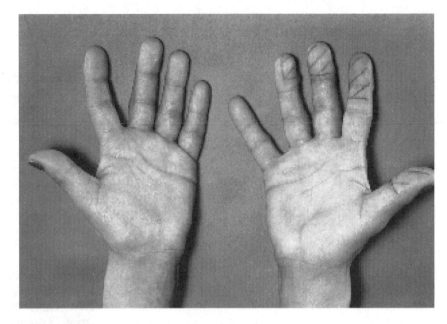

Fig. 10.2 The sensory loss in a median nerve lesion in the carpal tunnel. Sensory loss is limited to the tips of the fingers because the superficial palmar branch of the nerve does not travel through the carpal tunnel. The nail varnish indicates that these rather masculine looking hands belong to an acromegalic woman.

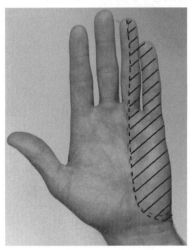

Fig. 10.3 The usual extent of altered sensation in an ulnar nerve lesion at the elbow.

Examination shows weakness of the dorsal interosseous and abductor digiti minimi muscles, and the first dorsal interosseous muscle between the index finger and thumb is often wasted (see Fig. 2.26, p. 20). Nerve conduction studies show conduction block in the ulnar nerve at the elbow. If the lesion continues to worsen after a month or two, or no signs of recovery are occurring by 12 weeks, surgery can be considered: simple decompression of the cubital canal or anterior transposition if the nerve recurrently dislocates. However, surgery is much less effective for ulnar than for median lesions.

Acute brachial neuritis (neuralgic amyotrophy)

This condition affects the individual nerves supplying shoulder girdle muscles and causes severe pain and weakness. It is usually misdiagnosed as an acute frozen shoulder and attributed to disease of the shoulder joint and surrounding tendons. The underlying cause of acute brachial neuritis is not known, although an infectious trigger is suspected. The patient complains of terrible pain in the shoulder which lasts between 3 days and 3 weeks. Then, as this pain subsides, weakness of shoulder abduction is noticed and the deltoid muscle subsequently wastes. Other muscles in the shoulder girdle or arm can be affected too. Supraspinatus (0–15° of shoulder abduction), infraspinatus (external rotation at the shoulder), and the long finger and thumb flexors are most commonly affected. Patients should be reassured that the condition usually recovers spontaneously, although this may take many months. There is no specific treatment. Physiotherapy maintains shoulder joint mobility during the period of paralysis.

Causalgia and reflex sympathetic dystrophy

Traditionally these terms were used to describe the chronic burning pain set off by trauma to a limb. The continuous pain of causalgia is often accompanied by hyperalgesia, an exaggerated sensitivity to painful stimuli, or dysaesthesia, which is pain after light touch of the abnormal skin. Causalgic pain often follows nerve injury, and an identical pain may occur in polyneuropathy, particularly in diabetes mellitus.

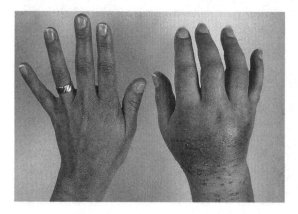

Fig. 10.4 Reflex sympathetic dystrophy affecting the right hand, showing swelling, discolouration, and skin changes.

Reflex sympathetic dystrophy involves a similar diffuse causalgic pain, not limited to the territory of a particular nerve, with associated oedema, altered skin temperature, and increased nail and hair growth of the limb (Fig. 10.4). Eventually dystrophic changes occur with indurated, sweaty, hairless skin and brittle deformities of the nails, known as Sudek's atrophy. Reflex sympathetic dystrophy can complicate a wide range of painful limb conditions, including trauma, surgery, arthritis, tenosynovitis, plexopathy, and radiculopathy, and can also occur after myocardial infarction or stroke when it is sometimes known as the shoulder–hand syndrome. Reliably effective treatment for reflex sympathetic dystrophy remains to be developed. Currently, causalgic pain is best treated with one of the drugs, amitryptiline, carbamazepine, or gabapentin.

Increasingly, the entities of causalgia and reflex sympathetic dystrophy are being described within the umbrella term of 'complex regional pain syndrome', mainly because of uncertainty about whether the sympathetic nervous system plays a pathophysiological role.

CASE 10.1 'BREATHLESSLY LOSING NERVES'

A 33-year-old woman with asthma developed worsening dyspnoea, purpura, and arthralgias. Interstitial infiltrates were noted on chest X-ray and her blood contained marked eosinophilia. A few weeks later electric shock pains radiated down the back of first one leg, and then a few days later down the other. She became asymmetrically weak below the knees with patchy numbness of the feet. An unpleasant burning pain developed in the little and ring fingers of her left hand, followed a few days later by similar pain in her thumb, index, and middle fingers on the right. Examination showed bilateral posterior tibial nerve lesions, with markedly worse weakness of ankle plantar flexion on the right side, and left ulnar and right median nerve lesions. After 6 months of steroid therapy her neurological signs had largely resolved and she was pleased by the improvement in her asthma although irritated by her cushingoid facial appearance.

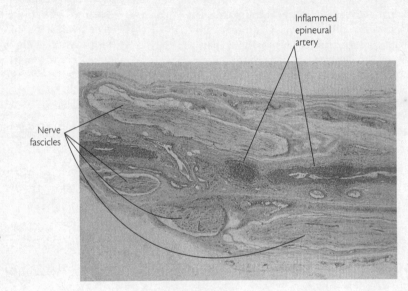

Inflammed epineural artery

Nerve fascicles

Fig. 10.5 Nerve biopsy (longitudinal section) in vasculitic mononeuritis multiplex showing an inflamed epineural artery, with a narrowed lumen due to a thickened vessel wall, surrounded by the nerve fascicles.

Comment

• This pattern of multiple individual peripheral nerve lesions is known as mononeuritis multiplex. It is most usually due to diabetes, and less often to vasculitis. If purely sensory nerves are affected, leprosy is likely in endemic areas.

• The subacute evolution with marked neuralgic pain in the territory of affected nerves in this patient pointed strongly to vasculitis. In vasculitis, the small blood vessels of peripheral nerves are occluded by inflammation of the vessel wall. If restricted to the peripheral nervous system, vasculitis may need to be diagnosed by biopsy of an affected sural nerve (Fig. 10.5).

• Sometimes the underlying cause is a systemic vasculitis as in this woman's Churg–Strauss syndrome, in Wegener's granulomatosis with granulomas of paranasal sinuses and lungs and glomerulonephritis, or in polyarteritis nodosa in which glomerulonephritis and bowel involvement are common. Less often vasculitis seems to be restricted to the peripheral nervous system.

• Vasculitic peripheral neuropathy is a medical emergency necessitating prompt diagnosis and steroid or cyclophosphamide treatment to prevent further peripheral nerve damage. If the vasculitis is quelled before irreversible and extensive nerve damage has occurred, good recovery can occur over subsequent months, as in this case.

CASE 10.2 'TOO MUCH IN THE PELVIS'

After mid-forceps delivery under general anaesthetic, a 30-year-old woman noticed right foot drop and numbness below mid-shin. These symptoms first became obvious on trying to walk a day or so later. Right ankle and toe dorsiflexion and ankle inversion were severely weakened but the ankle tendon reflex was preserved. The clinical diagnosis was of compression of the lumbosacral cord within the pelvis. This component of the lumbosacral plexus lies in front of the sacroiliac joint as it makes a contribution from lumbar nerve roots to the sacral plexus (Fig. 10.6). Characteristically such damage occurs after labour that has been protracted, involved a mid-pelvic forceps delivery, or involved cephalopelvic disproportion with compression by the infant's brow during an occiput anterior presentation. It usually recovers within 3 months, as it did in this case.

Comment

♦ The initial diagnostic suspicion of foot drop in such cases is usually of L5 or S1 root lesions due to prolapsed intravertebral disc, or a compressive common peroneal nerve palsy at the knee.

♦ Careful physical examination provides the clue to a lesion of the lumbosacral plexus by revealing a constellation of features which cannot be explained by damage to a single nerve root, or an individual peripheral nerve. For example, this patient had diminished sensation in the L4 and L5 dermatomes, and the associated weakness of ankle inversion (L4) meant that the foot drop could not be explained solely by a common peroneal nerve or L5 root lesion.

♦ Deficits due to temporary compression of healthy nerves recover spontaneously by remyelination in 8–12 weeks.

Fig. 10.6 Diagram of the lumbosacral plexus, showing the usual locations of lesions caused by different mechanical factors. (A) Lumbosacral cord compression at the pelvic brim by the fetal head or mid-pelvic forceps, causing maternal obstetric paralysis.
(B) Compression of the femoral nerve by surgical retractor blades in the gutter between the iliacus and psoas muscles. (C) Compression of the femoral nerve by haematoma within the iliacus fascia in patients with bleeding diatheses. (D) Lumbosacral trunk damage by traumatic fracture–dislocation of the sacroiliac joint.
(E) Angulation of the femoral nerve under the inguinal ligament during prolonged flexion and abduction of the hips in the lithotomy position.

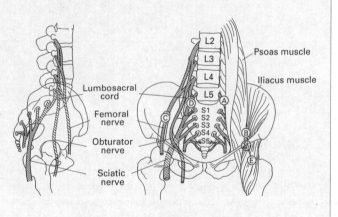

CHAPTER 11

Weakness V: generalized peripheral neuropathy

Polyneuropathy

Polyneuropathy affects all axons equally irrespective of whichever nerve they are in. If the neuropathy is due to axonal degeneration, the longest axons to the feet are affected first and most severely. If the neuropathy is due to demyelination it often affects the more proximal portions of nerves, and the nerve roots, so that proximal muscles as well as distal may be weak.

Polyneuropathy usually starts with tingling or numbness of the feet and fingers. Pinprick and touch sensation are lost in a 'glove and stocking' distribution (see Fig. 6.4, p. 47). Impaired joint position sensation may cause Rombergism and finger–nose ataxia. Weakness and wasting of muscles is mainly distal. Some or all of the tendon reflexes are lost. It is a good general rule that a patient is unlikely to have a polyneuropathy if the ankle jerks remain present.

Symptoms and signs in polyneuropathy are due to either axonal degeneration (Fig. 11.1(d)), demyelination (Fig. 11.1(b)), or focal conduction block (Fig. 11.1(c)). This important distinction is made by a combination of clinical and electrophysiological criteria. It has important implications for treatment and the potential for recovery.

Axonal degeneration polyneuropathy

Axonal degeneration polyneuropathy is due to exogenous toxins such as drugs (e.g. vincristine) or chemicals (e.g. glue solvents); to endogenous toxins (e.g. hyperglycaemia in diabetes mellitus); or may occur in ageing. It involves both the myelinated and unmyelinated sensory axons. Thus both myelinated (joint position and vibration) and unmyelinated (pain and temperature) sensations are lost equally. Involvement of unmyelinated autonomic axons causes a dry, warm foot. The distal

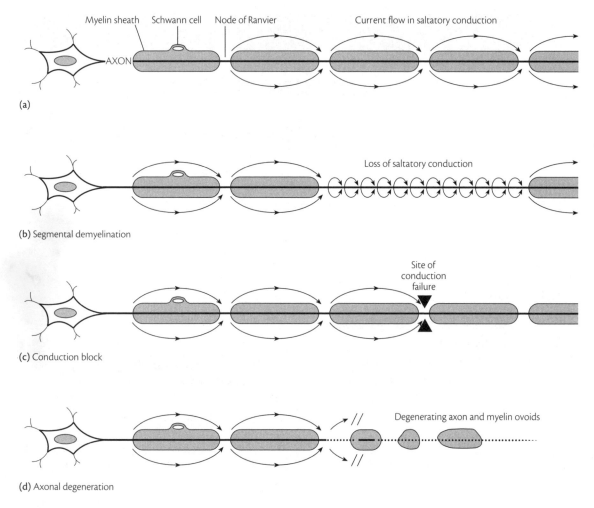

Fig. 11.1 Schematic illustration of axonal impulse conduction in (a) normal axon, (b) segmental demyelination after repopulation of the demyelinated segment of axon with sodium channels, (c) conduction block due to a local blocking factor or acute segmental demyelination, and (d) Wallerian axonal degeneration.

muscles are not only weak but waste markedly because of denervation. Although axonal degeneration polyneuropathy is generally less severe than demyelinating neuropathy, and develops more slowly, it rarely recovers well, even if the toxic cause is removed.

Demyelinating polyneuropathy

Demyelinating polyneuropathy does not involve the unmyelinated axons that subserve pain and temperature sensations or the autonomic fibres. Thus, joint position and vibration sensations may be markedly impaired but the pinprick and temperature senses remain relatively normal. Demyelinating neuropathy usually causes much more severe muscle weakness

than axonal degeneration polyneuropathy. This often includes the proximal muscles because the proximal nerve segments and nerve roots are affected. The degree of muscle wasting is usually less in demyelination because the axons remain in continuity with the muscle. The weakness results from blockage of impulse conduction in demyelinated segments. Demyelinating neuropathy is either due to a genetic abnormality of myelination (known as Charcot–Marie–Tooth disease or hereditary motor and sensory neuropathy (see Chapter 30)) or to an acquired abnormality of peripheral nerve myelination which is probably immunologically mediated. These acquired disorders can be acute, known as Guillain–Barré syndrome, or chronic known as chronic inflammatory demyelinating polyneuropathy. In areas where diphtheria is endemic, diphtheria toxin causes a severe generalized demyelinating polyneuropathy starting in the bulbar muscles. Demyelinating neuropathy can recover completely in a matter of months because remyelination occurs over 6–10 weeks after treating the immune or infective cause.

Nerve conduction studies

Nerve conduction studies can determine whether peripheral neuropathy is present, and if so whether it is demyelinating or axonal. It also proves the presence of a focal compressive neuropathy (Chapter 10). Measurements of sensory nerve action potentials and motor conduction velocity can be made.

Sensory nerve action potential (SNAP)

Peripheral sensory nerves are electrically stimulated and the afferent volley is measured proximally (Fig. 11.2). Small or absent SNAPs provide objective evidence for neuropathy, be it due to axonal degeneration or demyelination. By contrast, when a focal sensory disturbance is due to a nerve root lesion or central nervous system demyelination, the SNAP is normal because the peripheral branch of the axon remains in contact with the cell body in the dorsal root ganglion.

Motor conduction velocity (MCV)

An electromyographic electrode records the action potentials from a muscle following electrical stimulation of its nerve supply (Fig. 11.3). The conduction velocity is calculated by comparing the latency of muscle activation after stimulation from two measured points (A and B) along the nerve. It is normally about 50 metres/second. Also, conduction block has occurred if the amplitude of the muscle action potential is less following stimulation of the more proximal point (A) than it is from the distal point (B) (Fig. 11.6). A demyelinating neuropathy is diagnosed by demonstrating slowed conduction velocity and/or conduction block. In an axonal degeneration neuropathy, the motor conduction velocity would remain reasonably normal, but the amplitude of the muscle response would be equally small after stimulation at points A and B.

Guillain–Barré syndrome (GBS)

This is an **acute demyelinating peripheral neuropathy** which usually recovers completely. It can affect any age. Most cases follow an upper respiratory tract or gastrointestinal infection, 1–3 weeks beforehand; hence it is also called **postinfectious polyneuritis**. Various infectious agents can trigger GBS, the most common

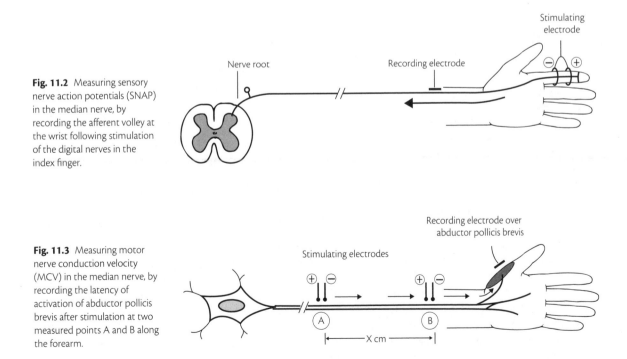

Fig. 11.2 Measuring sensory nerve action potentials (SNAP) in the median nerve, by recording the afferent volley at the wrist following stimulation of the digital nerves in the index finger.

Nerve root

Recording electrode

Stimulating electrode

Fig. 11.3 Measuring motor nerve conduction velocity (MCV) in the median nerve, by recording the latency of activation of abductor pollicis brevis after stimulation at two measured points A and B along the forearm.

Recording electrode over abductor pollicis brevis

Stimulating electrodes

A   B

X cm

being cytomegalovirus and *Campylobacter jejuni*. GBS can be precipitated by acute infection with HIV. Occasionally it complicates lymphoma or systemic lupus erythematosus.

The **pathogenesis** of the demyelination remains unknown. Possibly the infective agent evokes antibodies which cross-react with, or which precipitate cell-mediated attack upon, peripheral nerve myelin. Slowed nerve conduction velocities and conduction block prove that patchy segmental demyelination has occurred.

Clinical course

Weakness due to GBS worsens over 1–6 weeks, before plateauing for a few weeks and subsequently recovering over the next few months. The initial symptom is usually tingling and numbness in the toes and fingers. Sometimes leg weakness is noted first and there is little or no sensory disturbance. Arm weakness occurs next, often followed by life-threatening bulbar and respiratory muscle weakness. This **ascending paralysis** is symmetrical and the tendon reflexes are lost. Sensation is sometimes preserved despite complete paralysis. Instability of autonomic control occurs, probably due to oedema of nerve roots, and may cause wide blood pressure fluctuations, flushing attacks, and cardiac arrhythmias. Typically the spinal fluid protein is high with a normal cell count. A spinal cord lesion can be excluded because bladder and bowel control are not affected, and the plantar responses remain flexor.

Care of the paralysed patient

GBS and other generalized paralyses are dangerous for the following reasons:

1 **Respiratory muscle weakness**. This initially causes dyspnoea, and patients need to take frequent breaths whilst speaking. The vital capacity is reduced and should be measured regularly so as to detect deteriorating respiratory function. Endotracheal intubation and assisted ventilation, often via tracheostomy, are necessary when the blood oxygen saturation starts falling and there are significant respiratory symptoms. Respiratory failure is a significant risk when the vital capacity falls below 1 litre in adults. It is best to ventilate patients electively rather than awaiting a respiratory crisis. Before ventilation becomes necessary, it is worth discussing with the patient that, reassuringly, full recovery is likely to occur, but warning them that routine ventilation may be necessary for a few weeks.

2 **Bulbar muscle failure**. Dysphagia, a weak cough, and 'things going the wrong way' are signals of bulbar muscle weakness. They may occur even when respiratory muscle function remains good. It is just as important to carry out endotracheal intubation for bulbar muscle weakness as for respiratory muscle failure. This protects the airway and avoids the possibility of death by choking or inhalational pneumonia. **Nutrition** is maintained by a nasogastric feeding tube.

3 **Cardiac arrhythmias**. These are a major cause of death in GBS and require prompt anti-arrhythmic drug therapy or pacemaker insertion. The dysrhythmias result from autonomic instability.

4 **Pulmonary embolism**. Any paralysed patient is at risk of deep venous thrombosis and potentially fatal pulmonary embolism. This risk is minimized by low-dose subcutaneous heparin administration and elasticated stockings for as long as the patient remains paralysed.

A number of other measures are necessary to ensure survival and minimize permanent disability from an attack of GBS. **Chest infections** need antibiotic treatment and physiotherapy. Patients need to be turned regularly to avoid **bed sores**. Paralysed limbs should receive regular physiotherapy to prevent permanent **contractures**. It is **psychologically distressing** to be paralysed and ventilated whilst fully conscious; anxiety can be offset by frequent explanation and reassurance, and by taking care not to talk across the patient as though they were unconscious.

Plasma exchange or intravenous immunoglobulin (IvIg) infusion

Each of these treatments reduces the severity of paralysis and promotes earlier recovery in GBS if given within the first 2 weeks after the onset of neurological symptoms. Their effectiveness suggests that plasma exchange removes pathogenic antibodies, or that IvIg neutralizes them. Steroid therapy does not help GBS. Although IvIg and plasma exchange reduce the severity of GBS, it is vital to remember that the patient's survival depends upon the general medical measures outlined above. About 5 per cent of GBS patients die and 15 per cent remain unable to walk independently a year later, despite optimal therapy.

Chronic inflammatory demyelinating polyneuropathy (CIDP)

This chronic demyelinating neuropathy improves considerably with immunosuppression and is an important cause of reversible disability in neurology. Clinically it resembles GBS, causing severe areflexia, limb weakness, and joint position sense loss. However, it rarely produces significant respiratory or bulbar muscle weakness. The crucial distinction is that CIDP worsens over more than 8 weeks, whereas GBS crests within 6 weeks. CIDP is sometimes associated with monoclonal paraproteins in the blood, which may possess antimyelin antibody activity. Although most patients with CIDP have a symmetric sensorimotor disorder, pure motor and pure sensory, and multifocal, variants also occur. CIDP usually improves markedly with steroids and plasma exchange or IvIg. It tends to be a lifelong disease and spontaneous remission is rare except in younger patients.

CASE 11.1 'NOT GUILLAIN–BARRÉ SYNDROME AFTER ALL'

An 82-year-old woman was admitted with 7 days of severe neck pain, deteriorating walking, and parasthesia and numbness of the legs. For 5 days passing urine had become difficult, and for 1 day her arms were weak, numb, and tingly. Examination showed quadriparesis and diminished pinprick sensation below the shoulders. Because the tendon reflexes were largely unobtainable, and the plantars unresponsive, a diagnosis of polyneuropathy due to Guillain–Barré syndrome was entertained. However, the prominent difficulty with sphincter control, and the unusual occurrence of neck pain raised the alternative diagnosis of cervical spinal cord compression. A myelogram showed a block in the upper thoracic and cervical extradural space (Fig. 11.4), which was explored urgently by the neurosurgeons. A staphylococcal spinal epidural abscess was drained, and she was treated with antibiotics. Although subsequently tetraplegic for 2 months, she later improved with rehabilitation. By 1 year her arm strength was adequate for a full range of everyday activities, she could walk with a frame, and do without a urinary catheter.

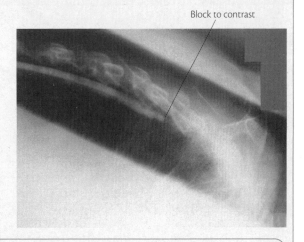

Block to contrast

Fig. 11.4 Cervical extradural spinal abscess. Lateral thoracic myelogram showing block to cranial flow of intrathecal contrast in the upper thoracic region due to an extradural mass.

Comment

♦ Acutely developing spinal cord lesions, most usually due to demyelination or acute myelitis, are the chief everyday differential diagnosis of acute polyneuritis, or GBS.

♦ In a patient developing urinary hesitancy or retention in the context of limb weakness, one should always be alert to spinal cord disease. Urinary hesitancy is a strong pointer to intraspinal disease, although sometimes it simply reflects the difficulty of micturating in the unfamiliar position of lying down, particularly in men.

♦ Although this woman was tetraplegic she never developed the respiratory failure that would have been expected had the diagnosis been one of severe GBS. The diaphragm, which was unaffected, is innervated by the phrenic nerve (C3 and C4 roots), which arose above the level of her epidural abscess.

♦ Speed is of the essence in diagnosing and treating compressive spinal cord lesions to minimize permanent long tract damage. This allows recovery, which is then measurable in months, and may be particularly slow in the elderly, although nonetheless valuable.

CASE 11.2 'A HEAVY WEDDING RING'

A woman in her 40s had slowly progressive weakness of the arms for more than 10 years. She had no tinglings or loss of sensation. She described very clearly that the first abnormality had been drop of the ring finger on the left (Fig. 11.5).

Later the right hand had weakened too. She had no pinch grip whatsoever and had to carry a short knitting needle in her handbag to insert through the eye of a Yale key so as to open her front door. Her stride lost spring on the left. A footdrop on the right made her a reluctant user of sensible lace-up flat shoes. Although the hand muscles had become relatively wasted, there was little or no wasting of the substantially weakened proximal arm, tibialis anterior, or gastrocnemius muscles. This combination of muscle weakness, but without wasting, allowed a clinical diagnosis of conduction block. In such circumstances the axon continues to contact the muscle fibre, thereby maintaining trophic influences, but nerve impulses are blocked from activating the muscle contraction. This diagnosis of multifocal motor neuropathy with conduction block was confirmed by motor nerve conduction studies (Fig. 11.6). Less than 2 days into her first course of high-dose intravenous immunoglobulin she called out in excitement 'look I haven't touched my face with my left hand for 2 years', as she raised her arm from her shoulder. A satisfactory level of arm power was restored by regular IvIg infusions, and she was particularly pleased to resume wearing stiletto heels for her daughter's wedding some months later.

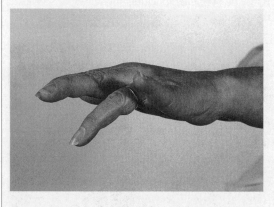

Fig. 11.5 Weakness of extension of a single finger: a common early symptom of multifocal motor neuropathy with conduction block.

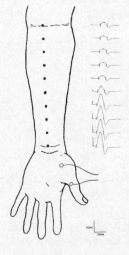

Fig. 11.6 Focal motor conduction block in a mid-forearm segment, demonstrated by inching the stimulating electrode along the median nerve in a patient with multifocal motor neuropathy with conduction block. The compound muscle action potential amplitudes from abductor pollicis brevis are shown to the right. Sensory conduction was normal throughout this same segment.

Comment

◆ This focal motor neuropathy with conduction block illustrates that focal blockage of impulse conduction can be a primary pathophysiological abnormality of peripheral nerve, without associated evidence of conduction slowing due to demyelination.

◆ Multifocal motor neuropathy was not recognized as a discrete diagnostic entity until the late twentieth century. Before that it was considered to be a slowly progressive, relatively benign, purely lower motor neuron form of motor neuron disease.

◆ High-dose IvIg is dramatically effective in such patients. Reversal of conduction block may improve weakness within 48 hours of first infusion.

◆ IvIg is used frequently to improve disabling neuromuscular disorders, apart from multifocal motor neuropathy: GBS, chronic inflammatory demyelinating polyneuropathy, and myasthenia gravis. Its mode of action remains unknown. Most likely is that it contains naturally occurring anti-idiotypes which neutralize pathogenic auto-antibodies causing the neuromuscular disease.

CHAPTER 12

Weakness VI: muscle disease

Muscle disease causes weakness, and sometimes wasting, of limb muscles that is predominantly proximal. There is no sensory loss. The reflexes are preserved unless muscle spindles have been damaged by severe inflammation or advanced wasting and fibrous replacement. Proximal leg muscle weakness is most obvious on trying to climb stairs or stand up from a chair. Proximal arm muscle weakness is evident on using the arm above the head, such as when hanging out washing.

If the weakness is due to muscle fibre damage the **creatine kinase** (**CK**) level is raised in the blood; a typical finding in polymyositis or muscular dystrophies. Needle **electromyography** (**EMG**) shows typical myopathic changes with motor unit potentials of small amplitude, and fibrillation potentials due to spontaneous discharges of individual muscle fibres.

The main aim of investigating muscle disease is to detect potentially treatable disorders:

- polymyositis (raised CK and ESR);
- myasthenia gravis (positive anti-acetylcholine receptor antibodies);

- iatrogenic steroid myopathy, and the rarer metabolic myopathies of thyrotoxicosis, Cushing's disease, or osteomalacia.

Much muscle disease is inherited **muscular dystrophy**, and accurate diagnosis permits genetic counselling or prenatal diagnosis of at-risk pregnancies.

The most important causes of myopathy are: polymyositis, muscular dystrophy, and myasthenia gravis.

Polymyositis

The muscle fibres are destroyed by inflammatory infiltrates; a cell-mediated immune reaction is probably responsible. Weakness usually progresses steadily over a few months. Aggressive forms can produce severe disability in only a few weeks. The muscles can be painful and tender. The CK and ESR are raised, the EMG myopathic and the diagnosis is proved by muscle biopsy (Fig. 12.1). Immunosuppression, generally using steroids, often allows substantial recovery of muscle function.

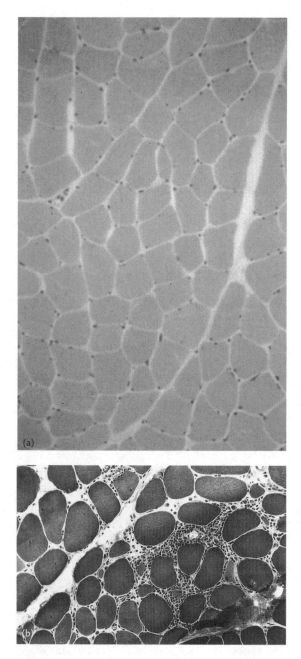

Fig. 12.1 Muscle biopsies: (a) normal, (b) polymyositis showing inflammatory infiltration between muscle fibres.

Other inflammatory myopathies include:

1 **Dermatomyositis**, with a violet (heliotrope) discolouration of the eyelids, and which may be associated with underlying tumours;

2 **Inclusion body myositis**, which tends to occur in the elderly and often involves dysphagia;

3 **Parasitic infestation** by the nematode *Trichinella spiralis* from undercooked pork in endemic countries. A puffy face, weakness of extraocular and bulbar muscles, and eosinophilia are typical.

Inherited muscular dystrophy

There are a wide variety of inherited muscular dystrophies. They range from those causing severe leg muscle weakness in childhood (such as X-linked Duchenne dystrophy in boys: see Chapter 30) to those which cause relatively mild weakness in middle age (such as autosomal recessive limb girdle dystrophies). Some dystrophies are diagnosable on clinical grounds because of their distinctive pattern of muscular involvement (e.g. autosomal dominant fascioscapulohumeral or scapuloperoneal dystrophies). The molecular genetic basis for these dystrophies is being elucidated and the mutations generally affect the proteins of the contractile process, the anchorage of these contractile proteins into the muscle cell membrane, or the intracellular energy providing pathways. Some genetically determined myopathies result from mutations of the mitochondrial genome, which is maternally inherited, and affect energy generation within muscle cells (Chapter 30). No curative treatment is yet available. The principle form of treatment consists of measures to improve mobility and hand use.

Myasthenia gravis

This is a rare autoimmune disease due to antibodies to the post-synaptic nicotinic acetylcholine receptor at the neuromuscular junction. These antibodies interfere with neuromuscular transmission by pharmacologically antagonizing acetylcholine binding to the receptor, and by reducing the numbers of available receptors. The diagnosis is proven by the presence of serum anti-acetylcholine receptor antibodies.

The muscles become weaker with use, a phenomenon known as **fatiguability**. This can show as bilateral eyelid drooping (ptosis) on prolonged television watching, a weak voice with a nasal escape due to pharyngeal weakness after prolonged talking, increasing leg weakness during walking, or inability to hold up the arms long enough to complete a hairdo.

Severe forms of myasthenia gravis may affect most of the striated muscles within the body leading to respiratory failure, inability to swallow, limb paralysis, and loss of eye movements. The survival of such patients depends upon assisted ventilation until treatment takes effect. Most patients have only minor symptoms, with intermittent drooping of the eyelids, diplopia, or difficulty in maintaining speed on long walks or during games lessons. Unfortunately some such patients are misdiagnosed as suffering from psychological disorders.

Neurological examination is entirely normal apart from the muscle weakness. No wasting occurs and the reflexes are preserved. You may be able to elicit fatiguable weakness by sustaining a movement for

5 Hz

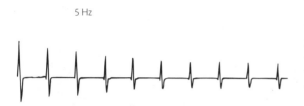

Fig. 12.2 Diagram illustrating how the compound muscle action potential amplitude progressively declines in size with repetitive nerve stimulation in myasthenia gravis.

a minute or so; for instance, diplopia may occur after prolonged lateral gaze, a nasal voice after counting, or ptosis after prolonged upgaze. Repetitive electrical stimulation of a peripheral nerve is diagnostic and shows progressive reduction in the evoked muscle action potential (Fig. 12.2).

Treatment is very effective in reducing or abolishing disability in patients with myasthenia gravis. **Anticholinesterase drugs** such as neostigmine or pyridostigmine prevent breakdown of acetylcholine in the synaptic cleft. As a result acetylcholine accumulates and stimulates the muscle receptors for longer. An injectable anticholinesterase, edrophonium or tensilon, reverses weakness within 45–90 seconds, and is used diagnostically as the **tensilon test**. Long-term **immunosuppression** with alternate-day steroids and azathioprine is very effective. Many younger adults with myasthenia gravis have an enlarged thymus gland with active lymphoid follicles, and **thymectomy** often allows recovery. Severe, life-threatening episodes of paralysis may be reversed by plasma exchange or intravenous immunoglobulin, to remove and neutralize pathogenic antibody respectively.

CHAPTER 13

Weakness of facial, swallowing, and breathing muscles

Facial weakness

Facial weakness is easily detected if unilateral. Lower motor neuron weakness is usually due to **Bell's palsy**. Upper motor neuron facial paralysis is usually due to stroke or tumour affecting the cerebral hemisphere. **Lower motor neuron** weakness involves all the musculature of one side of the face. In contrast, **upper motor neuron weakness** spares the forehead muscles so that the patient can 'raise your eyebrows' normally. Sometimes unilateral facial weakness is misinterpreted as dysphasia because it affects pronunciation of labial consonants ('p', 'b', 'm'). Doctors often fail to diagnose **bilateral facial weakness**, even though they notice that the patient appears to have an impassive face with a rather boring lack of facial expression. Inability to close the eyes tightly and bury the eyelashes, or blow out the cheeks without popping is the best clue to bilateral facial weakness. Bilateral facial weakness should raise the possibility of sarcoidosis.

Lower motor neuron lesions of the facial nerve within the skull also cause **loss of taste** on that side of the anterior two-thirds of the tongue due to involvement of the taste sensory fibres in the facial nerve. In practice, it is difficult to test taste reliably (sour, sweet, salt) on only one side of a protruded tongue. This limits the usefulness of testing taste in localizing lesions of the facial nerve.

Lower motor neuron facial paralysis

Bell's palsy

This is a common cause of unilateral lower motor neuron facial paralysis (Fig. 13.1). The cause of Bell's palsy is unknown. It may be a post-infectious phenomenon

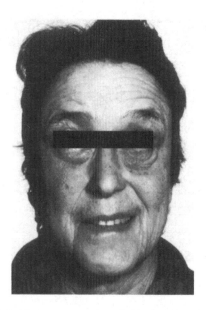

Fig. 13.1 A right lower motor neuron facial palsy with weakness of the corner of the mouth and the forehead.

which predominantly affects the nerve as it leaves the skull through the stylomastoid foramen. The facial weakness develops over 1–5 days and is often complete. There may be pain around the ear or a vague alteration in facial sensation during the first few days. Altered taste can occur, but is rarely noteworthy. To prevent drying and other corneal injury, lubricating eye drops may be necessary and the eyelids may be taped closed during sleep. Eighty per cent of patients recover completely within 2–3 months. A small, but significant number have permanent facial weakness, particularly diabetics and elderly patients. The risk of permanent weakness may be lessened by a short course of high-dose steroids if these are started within the first few days.

Other causes

One should always consider alternative causes for lower motor neuron facial palsy, particularly if it develops slowly or there are other associated neurological symptoms.

1 **Tumours** of the eighth nerve or skull base will show on MRI scanning. Deafness or palsies of other cranial nerves will be associated.

2 **Parotid gland** malignancies may be palpated; the facial nerve runs through this salivary gland.

3 **Sarcoidosis**; hilar lymphadenopathy will be shown on chest X-ray.

4 **Pontine lesions** of the facial nucleus due to demyelination or infarction. These are often associated with an ipsilateral VI nerve palsy causing loss of ocular abduction.

5 **Ramsay Hunt syndrome** due to herpes zoster infection of the geniculate ganglion produces severe facial palsy with a painful vesicular eruption on the palate and external auditory meatus. Parenteral acyclovir should be given promptly.

Bulbar palsy

Difficulty in swallowing (dysphagia), in articulating words (dysarthria), or in making sound (dysphonia) are the symptoms of weakness of the bulbar muscles. These are due to weakness of the pharyngeal and laryngeal muscles which receive motor innervation from the vagus nerve (X) and its laryngeal branches. A **unilateral palatal palsy** is due to a lower motor neuron lesion of the vagus nerve. It never results from an upper motor neuron lesion because the bulbar and tongue muscles receive bilateral upper motor neuron innervation. Thus, an **upper motor neuron lesion** must be bilateral before paralysis of the tongue and palate can occur, and the consequent paralysis will also be bilateral.

Palatal movement is examined by watching the soft palate rise as the patient says 'ah'; the uvula normally rises in the midline. A lower motor neuron lesion will paralyse the palate on the same side so it doesn't rise. The **gag reflex** is elicited by touching each side of the soft palate or posterior pharynx with an orange stick and watching the palate rise involuntarily. The afferent limb of the reflex is via the glossopharyngeal nerve (IX), the efferent via the vagus nerves. Patients with bilateral upper motor neuron lesions are incapable of voluntary palate movements, but the gag reflex will be present.

Most diseases causing bilateral upper or lower motor neuron palatal palsy also affect the tongue, and often the facial and mastication muscles too. The tongue should be inspected for wasting or fasciculation whilst it sits relaxed on the floor of the mouth (see Fig. 2.22, p. 17). When actively protruded most normal tongues appear to fasciculate. The power of the tongue muscle can be assessed by seeing whether it can be protruded to the normal extent, and whether it can waggle from side to side powerfully. A unilateral hypoglossal (XII) nerve palsy causes the tongue to deviate to the same side when protruded because of unopposed action to the tongue protrusion muscles on the normal side.

If bilateral paralysis of the palate and tongue muscles is due to a lower motor neuron disorder it is called a

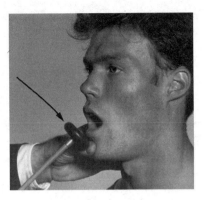

Fig. 13.2 Eliciting the jaw jerk. The patient's mouth should be half open.

bulbar palsy. If the paralysis is due to a bilateral upper motor neuron disorder it is called a pseudobulbar palsy.

Bulbar palsy is usually due to degeneration of lower motor neurons in motor neuron disease, to muscle weakness in myasthenia gravis, or as part of the polyneuropathy of Guillain–Barré syndrome. It carries the risk of sudden asphyxia from inhaling solids or of aspiration pneumonia.

Pseudobulbar palsy is usually due to bilateral cerebral hemisphere strokes, or to bilateral upper motor neuron degeneration in motor neuron disease. The tongue is spastic and tightly bunched, and the jaw jerk (Fig. 13.2) is brisk. Difficulty in containing the emotions is common in pseudobulbar palsy. Patients may become unduly tearful in response to rather trivial emotional stimuli encountered in films, stories, or conversation. When asked, patients with pseudobulbar palsy know that their tears or laughter are not true reflections of the depth of their emotional feelings.

Respiratory muscle failure

Respiratory muscle failure is generally due to weakness of the diaphragm rather than the intercostal muscles. It usually results from motor neuron disease affecting the phrenic nerve motor neurons (C3, C4 roots), from mononeuropathy or polyneuropathy affecting the phrenic nerve, or from muscle diseases such as myasthenia gravis.

Normally the diaphragm contracts and descends during the second half of inspiration. In turn, the abdominal wall normally moves outwards during the second half of inspiration so as to accommodate the diaphragm's descent (Fig. 13.3(a)). If the diaphragm is weak, the upper abdominal wall becomes sucked inwards under the rib cage during inspiration (Fig. 13.3(b)); whereas the weight of the liver helps its descent whilst standing. Thus, orthopnoea, or breathlessness on lying down, is the typical symptom of diaphragm weakness. This symptom is frequently misinterpreted as due to pulmonary oedema due to left heart failure. Diaphragm weakness can be proved by showing that the forced vital capacity is smaller when lying than when standing.

The motor neuron diseases

These are a group of diseases causing selective degeneration of the upper and/or lower motor neurons to the limb or bulbar muscles. Most types of motor neuron disease are quite rare. Both inherited and sporadic forms occur. They are most easily classified in terms of whether it is the lower, the upper, or both lower and upper motor neurons that are involved.

1 **Lower motor neuron forms**. The most notable is autosomal recessive **Werdnig–Hoffman disease**

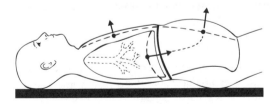

(a) Normal inspiration

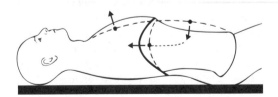

(b) Inspiration with a weak diaphragm

Fig. 13.3 Diagram illustrating: (a) how, during normal inspiration, the diaphragm moves downwards into the abdomen, with the resultant outward movement of the abdominal wall; (b) how, when the diaphragm is weak, the diaphragm is sucked upwards into the chest, with resultant indrawing of the abdominal wall, during inspiration.

which causes fatal limb and tongue paralysis in infants (Chapter 30, p. 177). The two main disorders affecting adults are sporadic spinal muscular atrophies, and an X-linked bulbospinal neuronopathy (Case 30.1, p. 180).

2 **Upper motor neuron involvement**. Limb spasticity due to purely upper motor neuron degeneration occurs in adults with **autosomal dominant hereditary spastic paraplegia** or the rare sporadic **primary lateral sclerosis**.

3 **Combined lower and upper motor neuron involvement**. Amyotrophic lateral sclerosis is the commonest and most severe type of motor neuron disease, and is usually fatal. It is often referred to simply as 'motor neuron disease', particularly by lay people.

Amyotrophic lateral sclerosis

Amyotrophic lateral sclerosis usually affects patients older than 50. Some younger cases do occur, particularly in the 5–10 per cent in whom it is autosomally dominantly inherited. It causes progressive muscle weakness and wasting, with prominent **fasciculation**, due to degeneration of lower motor neurons. Additional weakness and **spasticity** occur due to associated upper motor neuron degeneration. Patients do not have sensory symptoms, which if present would suggest a polyneuropathy rather than a motor neuron disease. Difficulties with micturition, defecation, or sexual function do not occur except simply as a consequence of immobility.

The first symptoms of amyotrophic lateral sclerosis usually start in one part of the body with speech or swallowing difficulty, weakness or wasting of a hand, or footdrop and leg weakness. The diagnosis is often not suspected until fasciculations appear in asymptomatic muscles in another limb, or the weakness is clearly spreading.

Examination typically shows a combination of upper motor neuron and lower motor neuron signs affecting the same muscle group. Examples include extensor plantars or sustained ankle clonus in a wasted fasciculating leg, a wasted fasciculating biceps muscle with a brisk tendon jerk, or a wasted fasciculating tongue with a brisk jaw jerk.

Electromyography shows denervation in muscles of all four limbs. Sensory and motor nerve conduction are normal, which excludes polyneuropathy. Patients affected solely by bulbar symptoms need an MRI to exclude structural brainstem disease. Those with lower motor neuron features in the arms and upper motor neuron features in the legs need MRI of the cervical spine to exclude a cervical spondylitic radiculomyolopathy.

Prognosis

Amyotrophic lateral sclerosis progresses over months or a few years to cause severe disability and eventually death. Leg paralysis requires a wheelchair. Arm paralysis makes it difficult to operate a wheelchair, and necessitates assistance with feeding, dressing, and grooming. Bulbar paralysis prevents swallowing of food and speaking, and leads to choking and inhalational pneumonia. Mental faculties are preserved, highlighting the distress of patients who are consciously becoming prisoners in bodies they can no longer move. There are no cures and no ways of arresting the inevitable deterioration in amyotrophic lateral sclerosis, although the drug riluzole may improve life expectancy slightly. It is bulbar paralysis, coupled with respiratory failure, that is the usual cause of death. This explains why the predominantly bulbar forms of amyotrophic lateral sclerosis have the poorest prognosis. In those with the bulbar onset, the median survival is approximately 20 months from the first symptoms, with only 5 per cent surviving for 5 years.

Telling patients about incurable disease

Amyotrophic lateral sclerosis is incurable and therefore the quality of pastoral care, and of palliative advice, are all-important. Patients should not be told the diagnosis until it is definite. Well-meaning relatives may try to prevent doctors from telling patients about the diagnosis of amyotrophic lateral sclerosis. But patients ultimately detect this **conspiracy of secrecy** at a time when death looms. That undermines trust and confidence just when these qualities are of inestimable value. In any case, the doctor's primary obligation is to respond to the wishes of the patient himself, and discussions with relatives should only be undertaken with the patient's express consent. Most patients want the disease to be named, and may even wish a frank discussion of prognosis, including how death is likely to occur. In answering such questions, one treads a narrow dividing line between brutal honesty and humane economy of truth. In any case, you should try and address the particular problems posed by that patient's own form of amyotrophic lateral sclerosis before they become upset by the summary generalizations so readily available nowadays in lay reference books and in journalism.

Anger is common in the months after being told about the diagnosis. This is particularly so in those too young to have become philosophical about their own mortality. However, anger should be seen as a natural phase through which patients with incurable disease pass before reaching the stages of bargaining, depression, and ultimate acceptance. Doctors may bear the brunt of this anger as though they were somehow responsible for the disease's occurrence. Only patience and understanding can preserve the doctor–patient relationship at such times, thereby laying the foundations of confidence which enable patients to trust their doctor's advice when miserable problems arise late in the disease.

Alleviating respiratory and bulbar muscle failure

Severe **dysphagia** can be treated effectively and discretely by percutaneous endoscopic gastrotomy via the abdominal wall. This avoids the need for a visible nasogastric tube. However, the patient or their spouse needs to have good hands and eyesight in order to change the nutrient bags at home.

Anarthric loss of speech can be offset to some extent by computer-assisted communication devices which are operated through a preserved motor function such as pressure, blowing, head-nodding, or blinking.

Decisions 'not to treat'

A particularly complex practical and ethical dilemma arises when making decisions about instituting assisted respiration in **respiratory muscle failure**. Very few patients would wish to preserve life by endotracheal intubation and ventilation when their body musculature has failed, and they know death is inevitable. Patients with distressing nocturnal breathlessness due to diaphragm weakness can be helped temporarily by continuous positive airways pressure delivered through facial mask devices. Once patients are aware that their substantial and disabling motor disability cannot be reversed, they may reach a joint decision with their relatives and the doctor 'not to treat' potentially fatal complications such as a chest infection. When they are immobile, dysphagic, unable to use their hands, can no longer talk, and are troubled by choking attacks and respiratory failure, most patients see death as a natural relief from distressing disability. If pressed, the doctor must be frank about what life under such circumstances involves, and be firm in agreeing a practical and humane plan of management. It is rare for a patient to wish for life to be prolonged beyond this uncomfortable and undignified stage.

Abnormal vision

Neurological abnormalities affecting the visual system produce two chief symptoms:

- **blurring** or loss of vision due to lesions of the sensory visual pathway,

- **diplopia** due to oculomotor abnormalities.

Loss or blurring of vision

A lesion can be localized to the optic nerve, optic chiasm, optic tract, optic radiation, or to the visual cortex by the pattern in which vision has been lost from the visual fields. These causes of visual loss should be distinguished from ocular abnormalities causing blurred vision, such as cataract, myopia and other refractive errors, glaucoma, retinal detachment, occlusion of the central retinal artery or vein.

Examining vision

There are four aspects to the visual sensory examination.

1 **Ophthalmoscopy** to detect primary ocular abnormalities such as cataract, due to raised intracranial pressure, or optic atrophy (see Chapter 2, p. 9).

2 **Visual acuity** measurement for each eye separately using a Snellen letter chart held at 6 metres. For a neurological examination patients should wear their spectacles. If the bottom line can be read, visual acuity is recorded as 6/4, 6/5, or 6/6 depending on the bottom line of that particular chart. If only the top letter can be read, vision is 6/60. If 6/60 cannot be read the chart should be moved closer by a metre at a time until the top letter is legible, recording 5/60, 4/60, 3/60, etc. If vision is worse than 1/60, the ability to count fingers at 1 metre or 0.5 metres should be tested, and finally the ability to perceive a torch flash. Any lesion affecting the representation of the fovea, whether in the optic nerve or visual cortex, will impair visual acuity.

3 **Pupil-light responses** to detect an afferent pupillary defect caused by an optic nerve lesion. The

pupil–light response is mediated via the brainstem and so it is not affected by lesions of the optic tract or visual cortex (see Chapter 2, p. 27).

4 **Visual field mapping** is the most sensitive way of localizing a lesion along the visual pathway. It is best to use a red pin, although fine finger movements provide an adequate stimulus for general screening purposes. The peripheral retina is specialized to detect movements and cannot resolve detail or colours.

Visual fields

You can compare the patient's visual field directly with your own by using a red pin in the following way. If you and the patient look directly into each others' eye and if you hold the pin exactly midway between, your visual fields will overlap and the pin will subtend identical angles in both your visual fields. If you move the red pin slowly in from the periphery, both you and the patient will see the pin head change from dark to red at about 35–45° from the midline. If the patient has a field loss they will not see the pin turn red until after the examiner. Red pin testing should be done separately for both eyes, particularly if lesions of the optic nerve or chiasm are suspected.

You can practise by mapping your blind spot, which corresponds to the optic nerve head (Fig. 14.1). Hold the pin half way between you so that it occludes the other person's pupil. Move it down just below the horizontal so that you can see the pupil. Then move the pin slowly laterally by about 20° and you will both see it disappear for a few centimetres within the blind spot (see Fig. 2.3, p. 8).

The main visual field abnormalities are:

1 **Blindness, or a central scotoma, of one eye** due to lesions of the optic nerve (Fig. 14.2(a)). These result from severe compression of the nerve by tumours, traumatic transection, infarction of the nerve, or demyelination in optic neuritis.

2 **Loss of a sector of the visual field in only one eye**. This is due to external, but incomplete, compression of the optic nerve, usually by a tumour arising in the optic nerve or in the bones of the optic foramen.

3 **Bitemporal hemianopia** due to compression of the decussating fibres of the optic chiasm by suprasellar extension of a pituitary tumour, or a craniopharyngioma (Fig. 14.2(b)). Bitemporal hemianopia can be relatively symptomless because the intact nasal field in one eye compensates for the corresponding blinded temporal field in the other eye.

4 **Homonymous hemianopia** is due to a lesion of the optic tract, optic radiation, or visual cortex on the opposite side (Fig. 14.2(c)). The usual causes are tumour, intracerebral haemorrhage, or cerebral infarction. Frequently this is noticed only because the patient repeatedly scrapes one side of their car whilst driving and hasn't seen the offending objects.

Having detected one of these visual field deficits, the next step is to arrange MRI of the brain and optic nerve

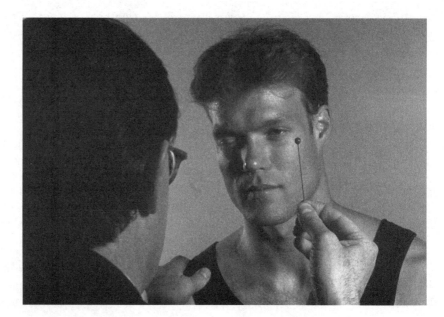

Fig. 14.1 Using a red pin to map the blind spot, which lies about 20° laterally, and just below the horizontal in each eye.

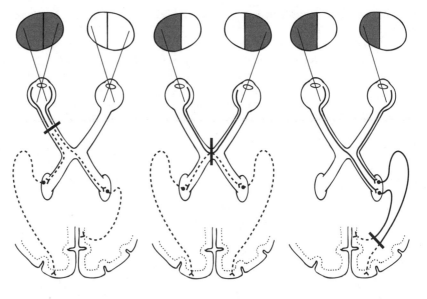

Fig. 14.2 The three main visual field abnormalities and the neuro-anatomical location of the responsible lesions.

(a) Unilateral optic nerve lesion   (b) Bitemporal hemianopia   (c) Homonymous hemianopia

to identify a structural lesion. Alternatively if optic neuritis is suspected, a visual evoked potential will show the unilateral delay, confirming a demyelinating lesion of the optic nerve. **Bilateral visual loss** should be investigated urgently. This is to detect a surgically removable pituitary tumour which would cause irrecoverable blindness if left to grow unchecked.

Optic neuritis

This is due to an attack of demyelination in one optic nerve. It can occur as an isolated phenomenon, or as part of multiple sclerosis. Over 1–4 days the patient notes blurred sight of one eye. This may produce a **central scotoma** (Fig. 14.3) or cause complete blindness of that eye. Often patients with optic neuritis notice pain on looking to the side. If the patch of demyelination affects the optic nerve at its junction with the eyeball, the optic disc may appear swollen, which is called **papillitis**. Papillitis can be distinguished from papilloedema because it is unilateral, and associated with

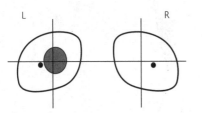

Fig. 14.3 The visual field loss in a central scotoma of the left eye.

profound loss of visual acuity. The visual loss of optic neuritis remains unchanged for 1–4 weeks before spontaneous recovery starts. Although vision usually recovers well, patients commonly have mild permanent deficits such as 'washed out' colour vision in that eye. The speed of recovery can be accelerated by a short course of steroids, but this makes no difference to the final extent of the recovery. The visual evoked potential is delayed from an eye affected by optic neuritis (see Fig. 8.12, p. 65).

An isolated attack of optic neuritis does not constitute a diagnosis of multiple sclerosis. After a single attack of optic neuritis approximately 40 per cent of patients go on to develop multiple sclerosis at some time, often many years later.

Pituitary tumours

These produce neurological symptoms when they compress the nervous system by extending upwards out of the pituitary fossa (Fig. 14.6). Such suprasellar extension may cause central forehead pain. Bitemporal hemianopia results from pressure upon those optic nerve fibres that are decussating within the optic chiasm (Fig. 14.2(b)). Bitemporal hemianopia is often asymptomatic, but patients may become aware that they cannot see the more distant object when they are converging their eyes to perform tasks like cutting finger nails, or threading a needle. Complete and permanent visual loss can occur if the tumour is not removed neurosurgically, usually by a trans-sphenoidal approach.

The various pituitary tumours produce different endocrinological syndromes. A basophil adenoma usually causes Cushing's disease. Acidophil adenoma causes acromegaly. Chromophobe adenomas secreting prolactin can cause galactorrhoea or may be relatively silent merely causing menstrual irregularities or diminished secondary sexual characteristics, such as reduced beard growth.

Diplopia and oculomotor disorders

Eye movement abnormalities are usually noted either because of '**double vision**' (**diplopia**) or because of a '**squint**' in which the two eyes fail to look in the same direction. These symptoms usually signify an abnormality affecting one of the three nerves that innervate the extraocular muscles that move each eye.

Sometimes horizontal diplopia or squints result from breakdown of a phoria (latent strabismus), usually temporarily, during infections or after a closed head injury. The movements of each eye are full when tested separately, but the eyes diverge when opened together.

Cranial nerve lesions

The oculomotor (III cranial) nerve

This innervates the medial, superior, and inferior rectus muscles and the inferior oblique muscle. Lesions cause paralysis of ocular adduction, up gaze, and down gaze. The nerve also innervates the levator palpebrae superioris muscle of the eyelid and provides parasympathetic constriction of the pupil. Thus, lesions lead to marked ptosis and a dilated pupil (see Fig. 2.15, p. 13). A third nerve palsy can result from tumour at any point along its course: carcinoma deposits affecting the nucleus in the midbrain, a malignant meningitis, by meningiomas in the cavernous sinus, and by tumour in the orbit or paranasal sinus. These can be detected by

MRI or cerebrospinal fluid cytology. But most commonly, third nerve palsies occur spontaneously in the elderly, in atherosclerosis, or in diabetes. Importantly, a third nerve palsy can result from compression by a circle of Willis aneurism arising from the posterior communicating artery which runs alongside the nerve, thereby signalling the potential for subarachnoid haemorrhage.

The abducens (VI cranial) nerve

Loss of ocular abduction occurs due to lateral rectus weakness (Fig. 14.4). This is less common than a third nerve palsy. Causes include tumour infiltrations and brainstem demyelination.

Trochlear (IV cranial nerve)

These palsies are rare and usually follow closed head injury. The paralysis affects downwards and inwards movements of the eye. It is best tested by asking the patient to 'look at the tip of your nose'. Correspondingly, the patient complains of diplopia when looking downwards to read or go downstairs.

Brainstem lesions

Gaze palsies are loss of the yoked movements which make each eye move equally in looking to one side, up, or down. Lateral gaze palsies result from lesions of the lateral gaze centre in the pons (Fig. 14.5). Vertical gaze palsies are due to lesions of the vertical gaze centres in the midbrain.

An **internuclear ophthalmoplegia** is due to a lesion of the medial longitudinal fasciculus in the brainstem, which prevents pontine lateral gaze centre signals from reaching the oculomotor nucleus (Fig. 14.5). This means that, although a gaze command causes abduction of one eye, the corresponding adduction of the other eye does not occur. Internuclear ophthalmoplegia is a characteristic feature of multiple sclerosis (Chapter 8, p. 64).

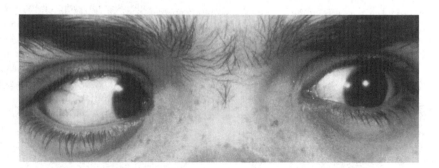

Fig. 14.4 A left sixth (abducens) nerve palsy causing reduced abduction of the left eye.

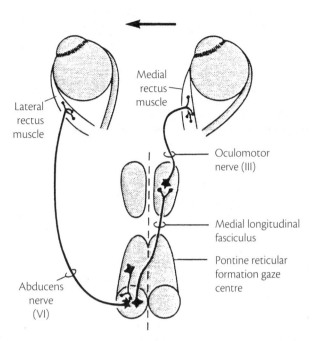

Fig. 14.5 Control of horizontal gaze movements, showing the connections between the lateral gaze centre in the pons, and the VI and III nerve nuclei responsible, respectively, for yoked abduction and adduction of both eyes.

CASE 14.1 'WHY DID HE WAIT SO LONG WITH FAILING VISION?'

Although presenting in his mid-60s this man's progressive loss of vision had started 15 years previously. It began on the left, remaining worse on that side. Initially he had been unable to see objects beyond his fixation point, for instance, locating his finger nail when using nail clippers. More recently he had become unable to read or appreciate television. Visual acuity was only 6/60 bilaterally, with a marked bitemporal hemianopia, bilaterally pale optic discs, and reduced pupil constriction to light. MRI showed a large pituitary tumour with suprasellar extension compressing the optic chiasm and adjacent hypothalamus (Fig. 14.6). The visual acuity improved rapidly to 6/12 bilaterally after trans-sphenoidal hypophysectomy.

Comment

- Visual acuity may improve quickly and surprisingly well after decompression of the optic chiasm.

- But vision can only recover if the optic nerve fibres have not been transected. Thus prompt investigation and treatment of bilateral visual failure is crucial.

- It is interesting why some patients with pituitary tumours take so long to seek medical advice. Perhaps the associated hypothalamic compression and hypopituitarism reduce motivation and concern.

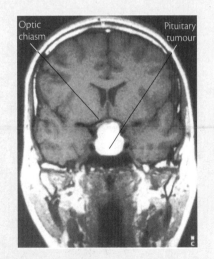

Fig. 14.6 Suprasellar extension of a prolactin-secreting pituitary adenoma compressing the optic chiasm to cause a bitemporal hemianopia.

Deafness

Deafness is usually caused by primary diseases of the middle ear such as otosclerosis, otitis media or trauma, or of the inner ear such as noise exposure, various genetic causes, congenital rubella, and age-related presbyacusis. Unilateral deafness is often not noticed unless patients find they are unable to hear the telephone earpiece with that ear. The main neurological cause of deafness is a tumour affecting the VIII cranial (auditory) nerve in its course between the brainstem and the internal auditory meatus. Partial deafness is a common sequel to bacterial meningitis or other infiltrating processes in the meninges surrounding the nerve.

Examining deafness

Impaired hearing is suspected when the patient is unable to hear a whisper in one ear. The principle aim is to determine whether it is **conductive deafness**, affecting mechanical transmission of sounds by the auditory ossicles in the middle ear, or **sensorineural deafness**, due to damage to the cochlea, or the auditory (VIII) nerve. This distinction is made using **Rinne's** and **Weber's** tests, which are best performed using a 512 Hz tuning fork (Table 15.1). You should try these two tests on yourself, and observe the effects of a temporary conduction deafness created by plugging your own external auditory meatus with a finger.

TABLE 15.1 Tests of hearing in conductive or sensorineural deafness

Stimulus	Conductive deafness	Sensorineural deafness	Normal hearing
Whisper	Reduced loudness	Reduced loudness	Normal
Weber's test	Louder on the deaf side	Louder on the good side	Equally loud in both ears
Rinne's test	Conduction in bone greater than in air	Conduction reduced in both bone and air	Conduction in air greater than in bone

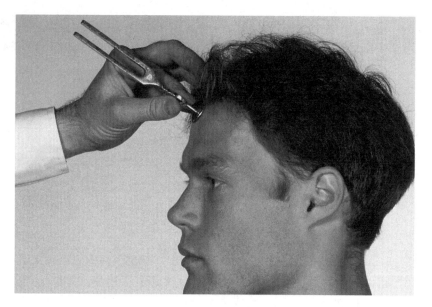

Fig. 15.1 Weber's test.

Weber's test

Put the vibrating tuning fork on the forehead and ask 'does it sound louder on one side or in the middle?' (Fig. 15.1). Normally it sounds equally loud in both ears. In sensorineural deafness it will sound louder on the **other side**. In conductive deafness it will sound louder on the **same side** because the vibrations are conducted to the inner ear through the skull bones.

Rinne's test

The loudness of the tuning fork is compared for bone and air conduction; normally air conduction is louder. Bone conduction is tested by applying the tuning fork to the mastoid process behind the ear, and air conduction by vibrating the prongs just in front of the pinna (Fig. 15.2). Bone conduction will be louder in conductive deafness. Both air and bone conduction are poor in sensorineural deafness. Confusion occasionally arises in sensorineural deafness because of bone conduction through the skull to the good ear on the other side, but this will be obvious from the results of Weber's test. In conductive deafness, you should inspect the ear drum with an auroscope.

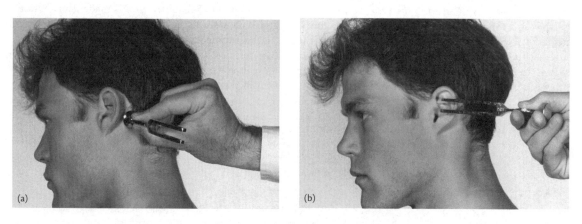

Fig. 15.2 Rinne's test comparing the loudness of (a) bone conduction; (b) air conduction.

Acoustic neuroma

This is a slow-growing tumour of the eighth nerve derived from Schwann cells. Small tumours within the mouth of the internal auditory meatus cause early sensorineural deafness. Tumours outside the internal auditory meatus, in the space known as the cerebellopontine angle, usually grow to a larger size before causing neurological symptoms. There may be facial weakness or loss of the corneal reflex response on the same side as an acoustic neuroma because the facial nerve (VII) also runs into the internal auditory meatus. Large tumours in the cerebellopontine angle may compress the cerebellar hemisphere causing ipsilateral limb ataxia, and may compress the pyramidal tract in the brainstem causing contralateral upper motor neuron weakness. Large acoustic neuromas can obstruct cerebrospinal fluid drainage from the IV ventricle causing hydrocephalus. MRI is very sensitive for detecting acoustic neuroma (Fig. 15.3) and for assessing any secondary effects such as brainstem distortion or hydrocephalus. Acoustic neuromas are usually removable surgically, although this runs a risk of permanent hearing loss due to VIII nerve damage.

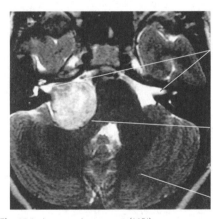

Fig. 15.3 An acoustic neuroma (MRI).

Internal auditory meati

Acoustic narcoma

Cerebellum

Neurofibromatosis

Multiple neurofibromas develop on peripheral or central nerves in this relatively common autosomal dominant condition. Many cases arise as new mutations. Acoustic neuromas are a common feature, and are often bilateral. Only rarely do neurofibromas cause mononeuropathy by nerve compression despite their frequent occurrence on peripheral nerves. The spinal cord, or individual nerve roots, may be compressed by neurofibromas arising on a nerve root within the spinal canal (see Fig. 8.13, p. 00) or an intervertebral exit foramen. The incidence of other central nervous system tumours is increased in neurofibromatosis. Gliomas and meningiomas occur and progressive blindness due to optic nerve glioma is relatively frequent.

Neurofibromatosis can be diagnosed by inspecting the body skin. Axillary freckling (more than six freckles per axilla) and *café au lait* patches are diagnostic (Fig. 15.4(a)). Multiple subcutaneous neurofibromas may be visible (Fig. 15.4(b)). If other diagnostic features of neurofibromatosis are not present, the diagnosis can be confirmed by taking a biopsy of a subcutaneous mass on the trunk.

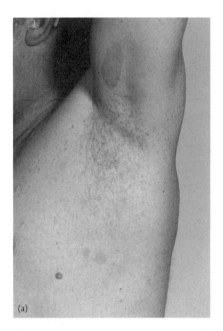

(a)

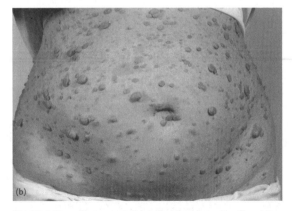

(b)

Fig. 15.4 Neurofibromatosis. (a) Axillary freckling and *café au lait* spots. Note the hearing aid. (b) Multiple subcutaneous neurofibromas.

CHAPTER 16

Dizziness, vertigo, and imbalance

Dizziness

Patients often complain of being 'dizzy'. It is important to establish whether they mean true vertigo, or merely a non-specific feeling of unsteadiness, with no illusion of movement, and no actual disability. True vertigo is an illusion of movement, usually of spinning round and round. To distinguish between vertigo and unsteadiness you should ask, accompanied by illustrative hand gestures 'do you feel as though you are going round and round (i.e. vertigo) or do you simply feel unsteady'. Non-specific unsteadiness rarely signifies a significant underlying disease; the symptom is often part of an anxiety state.

Vertigo

True rotatory vertigo is usually due to labyrinthine disease rather than neurological disease. The syndrome known as **vestibular neuronitis** or **acute labyrinthitis** may follow an upper respiratory tract infection. It involves abrupt onset of severe incapacitating rotatory vertigo, the worst of which subsides over a few days.

Ménière's disease causes recurrent attacks of rotatory vertigo accompanied by tinnitus (noise in the ears) and deafness. **Benign positional vertigo** involves acute vertigo and nystagmus when the head is turned into a particular position. These can be reproduced at the bedside, typically with a delay of a few seconds after the head is turned into a new position (Hallpike's manoeuvre). In practice, many patients with vertigo share features from these different syndromes. Drugs such as cinnarazine or beta-histidine are only partially effective in controlling symptoms.

Only uncommonly is vertigo a symptom of **neurological disease**. If so it is usually caused by brainstem demyelination in multiple sclerosis, or infarcts or tumours affecting the brainstem or cerebellum. Rotatory vertigo may be part of a migraine aura. Detailed examination of the cranial nerves, particularly eye movements, and cerebellar function is essential for excluding a neurological cause for vertigo. Patients with vertigo merit a brain scan if they have any other symptoms or signs suggestive of neurological disease, including headache.

Imbalance

A sense of **imbalance without vertigo** whilst walking is usually due to cerebellar or sensory ataxia. Patients generally describe having 'imbalance' rather than 'dizziness' and have experienced stumbling or falling. **Cerebellar ataxia** causes 'drunken walking', clumsy hands, dysarthria, and nystagmus. It may be due to tumours, demyelination, or degeneration of the cerebellum. **Sensory ataxia** also produces 'drunken walking', which is noticeably worse in the dark (Rombergism). It is usually due to peripheral neuropathy or disease of the dorsal columns of the spinal cord affecting proprioceptive afferent fibres.

Faintness

Syncope due to postural hypotension is covered in Chapter 21, as part of the differential diagnosis of blackouts and epilepsy. However, there are some patients with postural hypotension due to vasovagal attacks who do not lose consciousness and fall, but simply feel a mixture of being faint, unsteady, and sometimes vertiginous in the upright position.

Abnormalities of smell and taste

Taste loss

Most patients complaining of loss of taste have really lost their sense of smell. It is olfaction, rather than the taste buds on the tongue, that is responsible for most of our refined and interesting appreciation of flavour. Patients with loss of smell may complain that they have lost 'taste', but remain capable of identifying sweet, salt, or sour liquids with their tongues.

It is rare to encounter bilateral loss of taste sensation from the tongue due to trigeminal nerve (anterior two-thirds of tongue) or glossopharyngeal nerve (posterior one-third) lesions.

Testing olfaction

The most convenient way to test smell at the bedside is to ask the patient to tell you when they can smell your finger with their eyes closed, after you have pinched the peel of an orange, or put some scented soap on your finger. At the same time, you should block the other nostril with another finger. Specific smell-testing solutions such as cloves or peppermint are not neces-sary and rarely available. The patient does not need to identify the smell.

Anosmia

Unilateral anosmia is usually due to nasal cavity dis-ease. Occasionally it can be due to pressure on one olfactory tract by a frontal lobe meningioma; a physical sign that neurologists used to seek before the days of non-invasive brain scanning.

Bilateral anosmia usually follows head injuries or the common cold, and it may be permanent after either. Head trauma may shear off the 15–20 bundles of nerve fibres connecting the olfactory mucosa in the nasal cavity to the olfactory bulb sitting on the cribri-form plate above the nose just inside the skull. If the trauma also fractures the cribriform plate, and punc-tures the adjacent meninges, it can be associated with cerebrospinal fluid (CSF) leak, causing **CSF rhinor-rhoea**. This is potentially serious since it provides a por-tal of entry for bacteria and is a cause of recurrent meningitis. A suspected CSF leak should be investigated vigorously with a view to surgical repair so as to pre-vent this serious complication of recurrent meningitis.

Autonomic abnormalities

Autonomic failure

Symptoms of autonomic failure usually develop slowly. They many go unnoticed for years because of compensatory mechanisms. Persistent postural hypotension when standing leads to recurrent faintness, dizziness, episodes of vision draining away and blacking out, feelings of weakness, aching across the shoulders, or attacks of abrupt unconsciousness. Heavy meals, alcohol, some drugs, hot baths, or exercise can all provoke such symptoms. These symptoms are reversible by lying down. Autonomic dysfunction of the gut can cause attacks of diarrhoea at night, or pseudo-obstruction of the bowel. Autonomic denervation of the bladder and genitals makes voiding difficult and causes erectile impotence. Patients are often unaware that they have lost sweating, but direct questioning can reveal that their socks no longer become moist and smelly on a hot day, and that the finger skin has lost that moist adhesive quality required for effective grip-

ping of paper. Loss of the skin lubrication provided by the oily components of foot sweat may contribute to cracking, fissuring, and ulcer formation.

Autonomic hyperactivity

Although most autonomic disease represents a loss of function, attacks of autonomic overactivity can occur. The acute polyneuropathy of the Guillain–Barré syndrome can cause wide fluctuations in blood pressure and heart rate predisposing to cardiac arrhythmias, episodic skin flushing, and sweating disturbances. Autonomic dysreflexia occurs in paraplegic patients with high spinal cord lesions in whom bladder distension may lead to attacks of hypertension, bradycardia, and sweating.

Focal autonomic disorders

Focal damage to parts of the autonomic nervous system can lead to disorders such as Horner's syndrome of the eye (Fig. 2.14), due to interruption of the cervical sympathetic chain, or vasodilation and loss of sweating in a limb due to surgical sympathectomy.

Autonomic function testing

Although many complex laboratory tests have been described, the following are applicable to everyday practice.

Sweating

Loss of moistness from the palms and soles occurs in patients with peripheral neuropathies, such as diabetic, involving autonomic fibres. Sweating can be provoked by putting a hand in a plastic bag to prevent evaporation and warming it under a light for a few minutes.

Postural hypotension

Normally on standing the blood pressure is unchanged or rises slightly, and the pulse rate increases slightly. In autonomic failure the blood pressure falls and there is no compensatory tachycardia (Fig. 18.1). Normally, baseline blood pressure tends to fall slightly on repeated testing so it is advisable to measure blood pressure in the sequence lying–standing–lying and to compare the second pair of readings.

Sinus arrhythmia

Normally the heart rate increases during inspiration and decreases during expiration. This sinus arrhythmia is mediated by the vagus nerves. Disease shows itself as loss of variation in the RR interval of the electrocardiogram when recorded during deep breathing (Fig. 18.2).

Valsalva manoeuvre

Normally the blood pressure drops when one exhales forcibly against a closed glottis. Also, with the loss

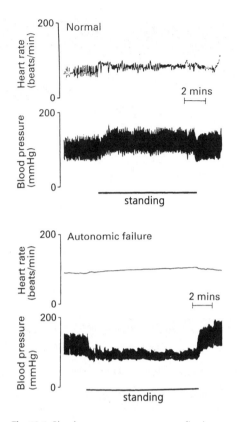

Fig. 18.1 Blood pressure responses to standing in a normal subject (top), and a patient with autonomic failure (bottom).

of venous return to the heart, the heart rate rises. Releasing this build-up of intrathoracic pressure leads to overshoot in the blood pressure because of continued sympathetic nervous system drive, and drop of the heart rate below its basal level due to baroreflex activation (Fig. 18.3). Autonomic failure abolishes this

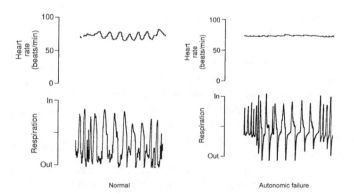

Fig. 18.2 Sinus arrhythmia of the cardiac rate during deep breathing in a normal subject (left) and its loss in a patient with autonomic failure (right).

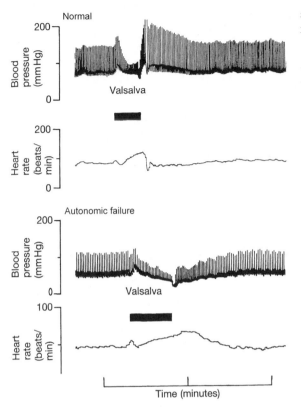

Fig. 18.3 Valsalva manoeuvre. The blood pressure and heart rate responses to exhaling against a closed glottis (▬▬), and then releasing the breath in a normal patient (top) and a patient with autonomic failure (bottom).

second blood pressure overshoot and the associated reflex bradycardia.

Some causes of generalized autonomic failure

Detectable abnormality of autonomic function can occur in a wide range of neurological and general medical disorders, although often it is asymptomatic. In everyday clinical practice, the common neurological diseases causing autonomic failure are diabetic poly-neuropathy and some cases of Parkinson's disease and related neurodegenerative disorders. Syncope should always provoke a review of a patient's medication for autonomic side-effects; this is particularly likely with some anti-hypertensive drugs. Vasovagal attacks, or simple faints, are an important differential diagnosis of blackouts, but are rarely due to identifiable neurological disease (see Chapter 21). Occasionally vasovagal syncope can be precipitated by hypersensitivity and compression of the carotid sinus, for instance, by a tight collar, in men standing to micturate, or in those with cough sufficient to cause a valsalva manoeuvre.

Facial pain

Pain in the face is common. It rarely heralds a medically serious disease, yet it causes considerable anguish and disability. It may present to neurologists, ear nose and throat surgeons, ophthalmologists, maxillo-facial surgeons, dentists, or psychiatrists. Accurate diagnosis is essential so that common diagnoses such as trigeminal neuralgia, sinusitis, or cluster headache can receive specific and effective treatment (Table 19.1).

Pain in the face can arise from disease of the cervical spine, eyes, or teeth. Pain from the ligaments, joints, or muscles of the upper **cervical spine** predominates in the neck and occiput, but can be referred to the forehead. It is often worse after energetic head movement. An **ocular** cause for pain is obvious in acute ophthalmological conditions such as the red eye associated with acute glaucoma. Refractive errors are probably an over-diagnosed explanation for forehead, eye, and temple pain, but spectacles may cure such pain in patients with astigmatism or hypermetropia who use their eyes intensely.

The unusual serious causes for facial pain include **tumours** of the paranasal sinuses, cavernous sinus, or secondary deposits in facial bones. Investigation of facial pain with CT scan of the facial bones and paranasal

TABLE 19.1	A list of facial pains
Common facial pains	
Atypical facial pain	
Trigeminal neuralgia	
Cluster headache	
Sinusitis	
Rarer facial pains	
Dental	
Temporomandibular joint dysfunction	
Secondary to cervical spine disease	
Ocular	
Tumours	

sinuses is particularly indicated if there is a neurological deficit, for instance, a numb half chin due to a mandibular lymphoma deposit infiltrating the alveolar nerve.

Atypical facial pain

Perhaps 50 per cent of patients have 'atypical facial pain' which is often associated with depression or anxiety states. Such pain usually consists of a rather non-specific ache, often imprecisely localized to the cheek, and it may vary in position or even change sides. Such pain sometimes responds well to antidepressant drugs such as amitriptyline, but it may become a chronic and intractable problem. It is important that one's first assessment of such patients clearly considers other identifiable and potentially treatable diagnoses. Because such patients often persuade surgeons to operate on their teeth, sinuses, or trigeminal nerves, eventually they may develop iatrogenic pains which further confuse the issue.

Trigeminal neuralgia

This is also known as *tic doloreux* because the intense momentary spasms of pain make the patient wince. Spasms of pain occur in the face, usually radiating from the corner of the mouth or from the gums towards the cheek and ear. The pain has a sudden electric-shock-like quality and shoots across the face. If patients complain merely of a steady ache, however intense, they are not suffering from true trigeminal neuralgia. Spasms of pain are set off by touching the face, shaving, cold winds, or by eating. The fear that such activities will provoke spasms may make patients unshaven, reclusive, or malnourished. The fear of pain may cause frank depression.

Facial sensation and the other cranial nerve functions are normal in trigeminal neuralgia. Trigeminal neuralgia usually occurs in the elderly. If trigeminal neuralgia occurs in young adults, multiple sclerosis should be suspected. If it occurs in association with deafness, facial weakness, or other abnormalities, a structural lesion of the brainstem should be sought such as an acoustic neuroma.

Carbamazepine prevents pain miraculously in most patients; treatment failure is usually due to underdosage. Sometimes it is caused by irritation of the nerve intracranially by tortuous brainstem blood arteries. Intractable cases may require surgical treatment, either by selective thermocoagulation of the trigeminal nerve roots, or by separation of the intracranial nerve root from any irritating blood vessels.

Cluster headache

Cluster headache consists of attacks of excruciating pain in one side of the face centred around the eye and lasting an hour or two at a time. It is also known as **migrainous neuralgia**. Typically it awakens the patient from sleep at around 2 a.m. and he may spontaneously say, 'it was so bad I felt like banging my head against the wall'. The pain is usually accompanied by reddening of the eye, tearing, and a blocked nostril on that side. Less often a Horner's syndrome occurs, with a droopy eyelid (ptosis) and pupil constriction which may become permanent in frequent sufferers. Clusters of attacks may occur every night for 1 or 2 months followed by remission for a few years. The pathophysiological explanation for the pain is unknown. Treatment of an individual attack is best achieved by self-administered injection or nasal spray of a triptan; oral treatment is too slow-acting to treat individual attacks. The following prophylactic drugs may be prescribed cautiously for a few months once a cluster of attacks has started: lithium carbonate (over-dosage can cause renal failure or encephalopathy), methysergide (prolonged usage can cause retroperitoneal fibrosis). A brief course of prednisolone, or inhaling pure oxygen may terminate refractory clusters.

Sinusitis

Pain is localized to the cheek in maxillary sinusitis, to the forehead in frontal sinusitis, and in the midline behind the nose in ethmoid and sphenoid sinusitis. Such pain is common in **acute sinusitis**. There is associated opacification of the sinuses on plain X-ray or CT scan, and antibiotic treatment is effective. Typically the pain of acute sinusitis throbs and may be lessened by ipsilateral carotid artery compression. There is often tenderness of the overlying skin. The pain subsides and recurs as the affected sinus empties and refills. Thus, frontal and ethmoid sinus pain is worse after sleeping and subsides on standing. In contrast maxillary and sphenoidal pain tends to worsen in mid-morning after a few hours of standing. Stooping, blowing the nose, or descending in an aircraft all exacerbate the pain of sinusitis.

It is uncertain whether facial pain also results from **chronic sinusitis** associated with mucosal thickening. Indeed, over-enthusiastic surgical treatment of such patients with sinus drainage procedures runs the risk of causing pain in its own right.

CASE 19.1 'PAY ATTENTION TO THE OCCUPATIONAL HISTORY'

A furniture maker of 50 developed unpleasant and worsening pain in his left forehead and side of his nose. Some weeks later he noted double vision when he tried to look down to read a book or walk down stairs. Examination showed a left trochlear nerve palsy, with paresis of the left eye on attempting to look at the tip of the nose. Over subsequent months much investigation tried to detect a tumour or an inflammatory lesion in the region of the left cavernous sinus or superior orbital fissure: CT, MRI, carotid angiogram, and spinal fluid examination were all normal. The working diagnosis was of cavernous sinus granuloma, a condition known as Tolosa–Hunt syndrome, and a trial of oral steroids was given. However, the expected improvement of pain did not occur. Left ptosis emerged, along with reduced left vertical and lateral eye movement reflecting new lesions of the oculomotor and abducens nerves. One year after initial presentation, further MRI scans showed bulging of the left cavernous sinus pointing to underlying tumour (Fig. 19.1).

Neurosurgical biopsy was considered to be both difficult and dangerous. So an ENT surgeon biopsied the adjacent ethmoid sinus. This revealed nasopharyngeal adenocarcinoma, an industrial disease of wood workers. Despite radiotherapy, which alleviated the pain considerably, the ocular motor abnormality worsened, culminating in complete left ophthalmoplegia. Eventually the patient died of this locally invasive cancer.

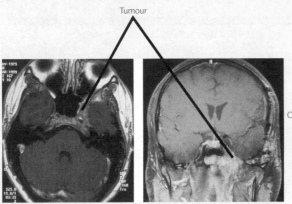

Fig. 19.1 Carcinoma infiltrating the left cavernous sinus. MRI enhanced with gadolinium: axial scan (left) showing tumour surrounding the carotid artery within the cavernous sinus, and coronal scan (right) showing tumour arising from the nasopharynx.

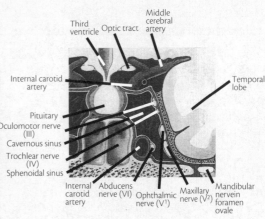

Fig. 19.2 Diagram through the cavernous sinus showing its close relationship to the various ocular motor nerves and branches of the trigeminal nerve.

Comment

- Pathology was suspected from the onset in the cavernous sinus given that the frontal and maxillary divisions of the trigeminal nerve, and the third, fourth, and sixth ocular motor nerves all run in or adjacent to it (Fig. 19.2).

- Infiltrating tumour must be considered seriously when patients develop severe, enduring and worsening pain in the territory of a peripheral or cranial nerve. Initially there may be little loss of the function of that nerve.

- Sometimes one first sees patients too early for investigations to have sufficient sensitivity to identify the structural abnormality responsible. If the undiagnosed patient is worsening, reinvestigation and assessment by specialists in related areas are the next moves.

- Definitive surgical excision is impossible of tumour infiltrating small inaccessible structures containing multiple nerves and blood vessels, such as the cavernous sinus.

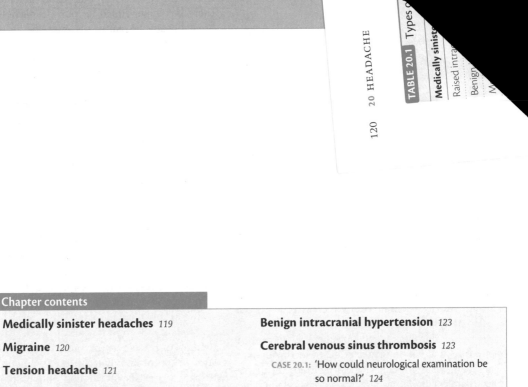

Headache must be diagnosed accurately. Medically sinister conditions need to be identified for specific and effective therapy to be prescribed.

More than 95 per cent of headache is due to two conditions without grave medical implications: tension headache and migraine. Nonetheless both can cause significant disability with time off work, and engender worry about serious diseases like a brain tumour. Table 20.1 lists the various types of headache.

Medically sinister headaches

Any of the following features should alert you to the possibility of a serious underlying cause for a patient's headache.

1 **Abrupt onset** occurs if a cerebral aneurism ruptures causing subarachnoid haemorrhage. Such patients recognize that the headache came on abruptly as though they had been 'kicked in the head' rather than developing gradually over a minute or so (Case 1.1). **Subarachnoid haemorrhage** may occur during exertion. However, repeated attacks of sudden headache at the moment of orgasm, with subsequent resolution, are usually due to 'benign coital cephalgia'.

2 **Headache on awakening** after lying down, or headache occurring **every day** without fail and worsening as the weeks go by, should make you suspect **raised intracranial pressure**. You should examine the fundi especially carefully for papilloedema. Such headaches in young women, who may be overweight and taking oral contraceptive tablets, are most likely to be due to **benign intracranial hypertension**.

3 **Focal neurology**. If a headache typical of raised intracranial pressure is coupled with symptoms or signs suggesting **focal neurological damage**, such as weakness,

... headache
... headaches (due to)
...ranial pressure (brain tumour)
...ntracranial hypertension
...eningitis
Subarachnoid haemorrhage
Temporal (giant cell) arteritis
Non-sinister headaches
Tension headache
Simple migraine (without aura)
Classical migraine (with aura)
Low-pressure lumbar puncture headache
Post-traumatic headache
Benign coital cephalgia

clumsiness, speech disorder, vertigo, or seizures, it points strongly to a **brain tumour**. Less frequently this combination signifies a focal cerebral infection with abscess, encephalitis, or tuberculoma. It is a good general rule that a brain scan is required in anyone who has both headache and a focal neurological disturbance unless this is obviously due to classical migraine.

4 **Meningism**. The headache of **meningitis** is associated with **photophobia** (dislike of bright lights) and relentlessly worsens over hours or days. Consciousness becomes impaired and **neck stiffness** can be elicited. Neck stiffness may also occur due to meningeal irritation in subarachnoid haemorrhage.

5 **Temporal (giant cell) arteritis** usually occurs in patients aged over 60 years with focal headache in one part of the head which is often too **tender** to touch or rest on the pillow. It is often associated with weight loss and claudication pain in the masseter muscles on chewing.

Migraine

There are two types of migraine: **simple (or common) migraine** in which there is no associated neurological disturbance (migraine 'without aura'), and **classical (or neurological) migraine** in which there is a preceding visual disturbance (migraine 'with aura'). Many patients have a mixture of both types.

An attack of migraine headache lasts between 3 hours and 3 days and usually does not occur more than once every 3–4 weeks. If the headache does not obey these time criteria, either it is probably not migrainous or there is a super-added tension headache—a so-called 'mixed headache' pattern. A migraine headache is usually thumping or throbbing in nature and often so severe that the patient has to lie down in a darkened room for the rest of the day. A migraine headache often starts in the forehead or occiput and is typically unilateral at least for the first few hours; indeed 'migraine' is linguistically derived from the Latin 'hemicrania'. However, bilateral headache does often occur in migraine. The diagnosis is suggested by at least one of the following: nausea, vomiting, photophobia, dislike of loud noise (phonophobia), or short-lived focal neurological disturbances.

Focal neurological disturbances, or **auras**, precede classical migraine, but not simple migraine. The commonest preceding disturbances are visual, with **photopsia** (coloured or flickering dots) in part or all of the visual field, or zig-zag lines called '**fortification spectra**' (because they resemble the ramparts of a medieval fort), or slowly moving visual **field deficits** such as scotomas or hemianopias. These visual symptoms last roughly 20 minutes, and precede the headache, tending to resolve at the same time as the headache starts. Less commonly the preceding neurological disturbance consists of tingling and numbness which march across the fingers of one hand, or across the face. Rarely temporary dysphasia, monoplegia, or hemiplegia may occur.

Migraine affects up to 5 per cent of the population at some time, usually starting in adolescence or early adulthood. A family history is common. It is commonest in women of reproductive age, often starting at the menarche, occurring premenstrually during the oestrogen withdrawal phase of the cycle, and ceasing at the menopause. Migraine headaches have an annoying habit of occurring when a period of stress has just finished; for instance, when the exams finish or the weekend is just starting. Wines, cheese, or chocolate may precipitate an attack and some patients can abolish attacks by dietary modification.

The pathophysiological explanation for migraine is not known. The traditional view is that it involves contraction, then distension, of abnormally reactive extracranial and/or intracranial blood vessels. Current theories of pathogenesis involve altered sensitivity of the trigeminovascular system of neurons, with a precipitating role for cortical spreading depression, which particularly explains the aura. Involvement of 5-hydroxytryptamine is suggested by the effectiveness of antagonist drugs such as methysergide, pizotifen, or the agonist triptans.

Occasionally **migrainous stroke** leaves a permanent neurological deficit after the aura. These strokes are about six times commoner than usual in sufferers from classical migraine. The risk of stroke in migraineurs is particularly influenced by smoking, oral contraceptive usage, and hypertension. Such migraineurs should be advised about this risk before prescription of the oral contraceptive. Indeed some doctors regard classical migraine as a contraindication to oral contraception.

Formal **treatment** is not necessary for many migraineurs. Attacks are often mild, infrequent, precipitated by avoidable foods, or resolve with **simple analgesics** and **anti-emetic** preparations. Those with frequent (more than 12/year), prolonged and disabling attacks benefit from daily prophylaxis using propranolol (avoid in asthmatics) or pizotifen (causes drowsiness and weight gain). Methysergide can be considered in refractory cases but carries the risk of retroperitoneal fibrosis and should never be given for more than 6–9 months at a time. Individual severe attacks can be treated with a **triptan** by mouth, or by self-administered injection or nasal spray if vomiting precludes swallowing a tablet. **Ergotamine** used to be prescribed for individual attacks, but dangerous vasoconstriction and gangrene could follow excessive use, and it is itself a cause of headache in those who habitually over-consume it.

Tension headache

This headache is as common as migraine. It is the main cause of **chronic daily headache**. It is distinguished from migraine by the lack of discrete attacks, and by its bilaterality. Tension headache occurs nearly every day for weeks or months on end. Its severity fluctuates so that patients often realize that a few hours have passed when it has been barely noticeable. Usually the headache is worse frontally, or occipitally, and it frequently encircles the entire head. The pain is often described as achy, pressing, or tight. Patients may volunteer that 'it is like a tight band (or hat) around my head'. Focal neurological disturbance, nausea and vomiting, or photophobia do not occur. Typically, simple analgesics such as aspirin or paracetamol are ineffective.

The pathophysiological mechanism of tension headache is not known. Its name is derived from the notion of chronic muscle tension with resultant impairment of blood supply to muscles and the scalp. It often occurs in young adults who are weighed down by the demands of young families and employment, and who

have stopped exercising regularly. A subgroup of patients have clear evidence of underlying depression with early morning waking, tearfulness, a sense of worthlessness, melancholy, weight and appetite fluctuation, or loss of libido. Some patients fear a brain tumour and this morbid anxiety may worsen their headache. Occasional patients will settle for nothing less than the reassurance of a (normal) brain scan.

Reassurance, resumption of regular exercise, or relaxation exercises are often effective in the milder cases, many of whom do not wish to consume regular medication. **Amitriptyline**, often in very low dosage, is usually effective whether or not there is a formal depressive disorder. It is best given in the evening so that its sedative side-effect merges with sleep. The patient may presume that, because an 'antidepressant drug' has been prescribed, the doctor regards them as being depressed and neurotic and is simply avoiding pointing this out. It is worth saying that 'amitriptyline is a drug which is normally used in depression, but which was found incidentally to have a very specific effect against tension headaches, which is why I'm recommending it to you'.

Temporal (giant cell) arteritis

Delay or misdiagnosis of temporal arteritis can allow the feared complication of **permanent loss of sight** in one eye to develop due to occlusion of the ophthalmic artery. As a general rule **both the patient and their erythrocyte sedimentation rate (ESR) are over 60**; although occasional exceptions do occur. Patients report intense focal headache, usually in the temporal or occipital region, and note exquisite scalp tenderness especially on resting their head on the pillow. They have often lost weight and note early morning aching of their limb or trunk muscles due to the associated condition of **polymyalgia rheumatica**. **Jaw claudication** may occur on chewing, with aching of the masseter or temporalis muscles; this is a very suggestive symptom of temporal arteritis. The temporal arteries are typically tender, swollen, and non-pulsatile. It is easiest to start palpation by finding the pulsatile segment of the artery just in front of the ear, and then following it distally into the hairline (Fig. 20.1).

The ESR is usually greatly elevated to over 100 mm/hour. The diagnosis is proved by temporal artery biopsy, which shows arteritis and giant cells (Fig. 20.2).

Immediate steroid therapy prevents extension to the ophthalmic artery. Steroids are usually curative but may need to be continued for 2 years or more, with the

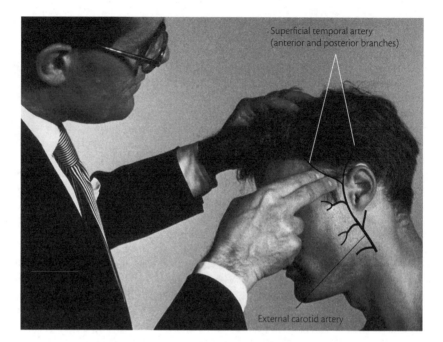

Fig. 20.1 How to palpate the temporal artery.

attendant risks of susceptibility to infection, proximal myopathy, and osteoporotic vertebral collapse. Indeed intravenous hydrocortisone is recommended immediately the diagnosis is seriously suspected, so as to forestall visual loss. The diagnostic temporal artery biopsy can be undertaken within the next day or two after starting steroids.

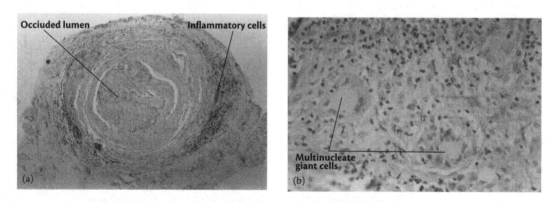

Fig. 20.2 Temporal (giant cell) arteritis. (a) Transverse section of temporal artery showing disruption of the vessel wall, infiltration with cells; and obliteration of the lumen; (b) mutinucleate giant cells.

Benign intracranial hypertension

This usually occurs in young women who may be **obese**, taking the **oral contraceptive tablet**, or using long-term **tetracyclines** to prevent acne. Over a few months, daily headache worsens. It has the characteristics of raised intracranial pressure: worse on awakening and worsened by coughing or straining. Papilloedema is present. Initially a cerebral tumour may be suspected, but focal abnormalities are not present on examination and the MRI scan is normal; hence it is also known as **pseudotumour cerebri**. Armed with the knowledge that the brain scan is normal, you can safely prove the diagnosis by measuring the raised cerebrospinal fluid (CSF) pressure (>20 cm H_2O) at lumbar puncture. The **cause** of benign intracranial hypertension is unknown but involves overproduction or under-resorption of CSF.

Benign intracranial hypertension often remits spontaneously after advice about dieting and stopping oral contraceptive or tetracycline medication. In many patients the symptoms remain stable and do not threaten vision; acetazolamide or thiazide diuretics, and analgesics may be helpful. The best way to monitor the condition is by repeated measurement of the visual acuity and of the size of the blind spots. These reflect the degree of papilloedema and hence the spinal fluid pressure. Some patients develop chronically elevated CSF pressure, which causes **optic nerve damage**; this is heralded by enlarging blind spots, decreasing visual acuity, and generally constricted visual fields. For such patients it is currently recommended that surgical fenestration of the optic nerve or ventriculo-peritoneal shunting are carried out to promote CSF drainage and protect the optic nerves from damage.

Cerebral venous sinus thrombosis

Occasionally a similar syndrome occurs as a result of cerebral venous sinus thrombosis particularly in those with inherited coagulation abnormalities (such as factor V Leiden) or using oral contraceptives. The thrombosed venous sinus is easily visualized on MRI (Fig. 20.3). But usually sagittal sinus thrombosis is of more abrupt onset with impaired consciousness, seizures, and hemiparesis or aphasia; many patients die or develop permanent neurological deficits. Apart from those with coagulation disorders, it may also occur in pregnancy, with middle ear infection, or in grossly dehydrated and cachectic patients. Welcome recovery may occur when anticoagulation is started.

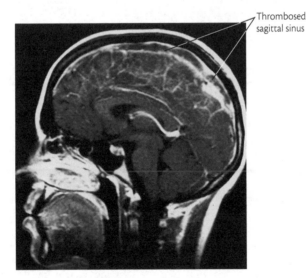

Thrombosed sagittal sinus

Fig. 20.3 Sagittal venous sinus thrombosis (MRI scan).

CASE 20.1 'HOW COULD NEUROLOGICAL EXAMINATION BE SO NORMAL?'

Every 3 months or so since her menarche, a 30-year-old woman had left-sided 'migraine' headaches associated with vomiting and imbalance. Each resolved within 2–3 days. For 2 or 3 years she also had milder background headache 'like a clamp' present all day on most, but not all days. Neurological examination was completely normal. A mixed headache picture was diagnosed, with long-standing migraine attacks, and the more recent development of muscle tension headache. However, because of the complaint that she always felt slightly 'off balance' a brain scan was arranged (Fig. 20.4). Surprisingly this showed a huge cerebellar tumour, typical of a cerebellar haemangioblastoma. Before referring her to a neurosurgeon, who later excised the tumour to confirm the diagnosis, the patient was re-examined neurologically in some detail. Once again, no abnormal physical signs could be detected. Under close questioning she did recall that her father had had 'blood vessel tumours in his eyes'.

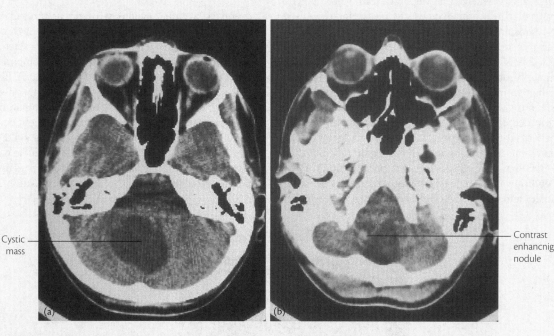

Cystic mass

Contrast enhancnig nodule

Fig. 20.4 Cerebellar haemangioblastoma. CT scan unenhanced (a) showing a large cystic mass in the posterior fossa which when contrast enhanced (b) was typical of haemangioblastoma.

Comment

- This patient's imbalance was due to a posterior cranial fossa tumour. It remained uncertain whether her headache was due to the tumour or whether it was simply a normal tension headache.

- When to arrange a brain scan in those patients seemingly suffering from muscle tension headache? Do so if there are physical signs, or an additional symptom, suggestive of a structural abnormality affecting the brain.

- This woman had von Hippel–Lindau disease. It is an autosomal dominant condition due to mutation of a tumour suppressor gene. This predisposes to cerebellar and spinal hemangioblastomas, retinal angiomas, phaeochromocytoma, and also to renal carcinoma, which was later detected in her.

CASE 20.2 'I'M AFRAID I'VE GOT A HEADACHE'

At the moment of orgasm a man in his 60s developed severe occipital headache which persisted throughout the night. He was referred the very next morning. Although the story was compatible with a diagnosis of benign coital cephalgia, or sex headache, it is unusual for this first to occur at this age, and for the headache to last so long afterwards. Cerebral angiography revealed a cerebral aneurism which was obliterated endovascularly by interventional angiography (Fig. 20.5). Knowing that the threat of aneurismal rupture was now behind him, he was able to return to his normal life.

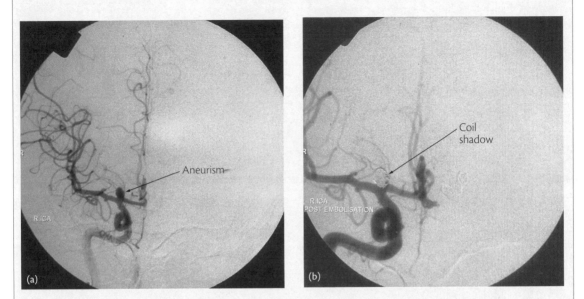

Fig. 20.5 Cerebral aneurism shown at carotid angiography before (a) and after (b) obliteration by endovascular coiling.

Comment

- The diagnosis of benign coital cephalgia can only be made with confidence after repeated typical occurrences, without any sinister outcome.

- Exertion or excitement are well-recognized precipitators of haemorrhage from cerebral aneurisms.

- Interventional radiological obliteration of cerebral aneurisms is replacing open neurosurgical clipping. It avoids damage to adjacent brain during neurosurgical manipulation. Rebleeds can be avoided because it can be performed early. It avoids the risk of post-craniotomy epilepsy and the associated bar from driving.

CHAPTER 21

Epilepsy and blackouts

Blackouts and funny turns

The three commonest causes of blackouts are:

1 epilepsy,

2 vasovagal attacks (simple faints),

3 cardiac arrhythmias.

The differences between these are considered below. Although seizures sometimes occur in **hyperventilation** or **hypoglycaemia**, unconsciousness due to these conditions is usually not epileptic. Transient cerebral ischaemic attacks due to emboli almost never produce unconsciousness. Rarely, a migraine aura can involve unconsciousness, so-called basilar migraine.

Many patients complain of **funny turns**, in which the period of unconsciousness is not clearly definable. Sometimes these reflect a period of being flustered due to anxiety, possibly with an element of hyperventilation. Introspective patients may be concerned to realize they have no conscious memory of a routine activity, such as driving a familiar route without incident. Psychologically determined **fugue states** or amnesias can occur, and are often characterized by the completely featureless nature of the history that is obtainable. **Transient global amnesia** attacks last a few hours, in which patients undertake their lives seemingly normally, only to have no subsequent memory of that period of time.

The history is crucial and yet a patient cannot describe what they did whilst unconscious. If possible, you should interview an **eyewitness** to determine whether a **convulsion** occurred. Furthermore, a witness may have taken the pulse, thereby diagnosing (or excluding) a cardiac arrhythmia.

Diagnosing an epileptic seizure

An eyewitness description of a typical **convulsion** is diagnostic. **Tonic** convulsions involve generalized stiffening of the limbs. **Clonic** convulsions are coarse, powerful, and repetitive shakings of the limbs. Most seizures are tonic, before becoming clonic. A seizure may be **focal** (affecting one limb, or one side of the face) or **generalized** (affecting both sides of the body equally). It lasts a minute or so usually.

If a blackout has not been witnessed, one or more of the following features point strongly to a diagnosis of epilepsy (Table 21.1).

1 **Postictal confusion** lasting 5–20 minutes. In contrast, patients with vasovagal attacks or cardiac arrhythmias usually become fully orientated within a few moments of waking up. Beware of the patient who has simply fainted, but suffers concussion after banging their head on the pavement.

2 **Incontinence of urine**.

3 **Biting the tongue** or cheek. But occasionally you may be confused by a patient who has fainted in the bathroom and bitten their tongue as a result of catching their chin on the sink whilst falling.

4 **Failure to remember the onset of the blackout**. In contrast, patients with vasovagal or cardiogenic blackouts usually have a clear recollection of 'fading away' at the onset.

5 **Sudden absence attacks** as though the patient has 'turned off' and lost contact with their surroundings. In children these are usually due to petit mal epi-

lepsy. In adults, and some children, they are due to temporal lobe epileptic discharges which may be associated with automatic behaviours, head and eye deviations, or lip smacking and chewing movements. Of course many of us have momentary attacks of inattention, when our mind wanders, but we remain responsive to outside stimuli.

6 **Auras** or stereotyped hallucinations are typical of temporal lobe epileptic discharges. Uncinate hallucinations involve a strange smell or taste, often resembling burning rubber. *Déja vu* is a feeling of intense familiarity with an unfamiliar environment; *jamais vu* is the opposite. **Macropsia** makes a visual scene seem closer and bigger than it really is; micropsia is the opposite.

A blackout should not be diagnosed as epileptic unless there is firm evidence of at least one of these features or a definite convulsion has been observed. Otherwise, a patient wrongly diagnosed as epileptic will be vulnerable to social and employment stigmas, driving restrictions, and unjustified prescription of anticonvulsant drugs.

Types of epilepsy

An epileptic attack is '**an electrical brain-storm**'. This can be recorded by an **electro-encephalogram (EEG)** recorded from an array of electrodes covering the scalp. A **spike and slow-wave discharge** is the only EEG abnormality which is absolutely diagnostic of an epileptic disturbance (Fig. 21.1). A routine EEG recording period of an hour or so is very unlikely to capture an attack in patients with intermittent grand mal or focal epileptic attacks. For this reason, particularly in adults, a routine EEG rarely helps to make the diagnosis of epilepsy; an eyewitness account or critical history taking are much more valuable. However, the EEG is often diagnostic in children with petit mal epilepsy causing absence attacks. In them voluntary overbreathing may provoke typical 3/second slow-wave and spike discharges often without an observable attack.

It is easiest to think of seizures as being either **primarily generalized**, **focal**, or **secondarily generalized** from a focus. In reality there are numerous epilepsy

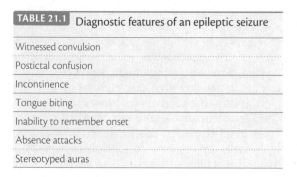

TABLE 21.1 Diagnostic features of an epileptic seizure

Witnessed convulsion
Postictal confusion
Incontinence
Tongue biting
Inability to remember onset
Absence attacks
Stereotyped auras

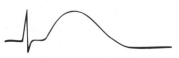

Fig. 21.1 An epileptic spike and slow-wave discharge.

syndromes, with their classification being determined increasingly by the underlying genetic abnormality, for instance, mutations in genes for neuronal ion channels.

Primarily generalized epilepsies

The epileptic discharge occurs simultaneously throughout the brain. The commonest type is 3/sec slow-wave and spike discharge in childhood absence epilepsy (Fig. 21.2). Parents or teachers observe absence, or **petit mal**, attacks in which the child repeatedly switches off for a moment or two, perhaps blinking vacantly, but does not convulse and usually does not fall down. As the attack finishes the child resumes their activities and may be unaware that anything has happened. Sometimes the attacks themselves have not been observed, but deteriorating school performance is noted. You may be able to provoke an attack in the clinic by asking the child to hyperventilate in front of you. Children usually grow out of petit mal epilepsy in their late teens.

Another type of primarily generalized epilepsy is **juvenile myoclonic epilepsy**. Children and adolescents have attacks of absence associated with sudden myoclonic jerkings, which consist of shock-like twitches of the limbs. Grand mal convulsions occur too, often soon after awakening.

Both childhood absence epilepsy and juvenile myoclonic epilepsy are genetically determined. **Sodium valproate** is usually very effective as treatment, with lamotrigine as an alternative.

Focal epilepsies

Focal epileptic attacks arise from brain abnormalities such as tumours, infections, infarcts, after head injuries, or from hippocampal sclerosis due to frequent childhood febrile convulsions. Such patients must be investigated with brain **MRI** so that underlying focal abnormalities can be treated. In some younger patients with frequent seizures unresponsive to standard anticonvulsant drugs, the epilepsy may be improved or even abolished by **surgical resection** of hippocampal sclerosis. Only rarely can you capture focal spike discharges on a routine EEG (Fig. 21.3).

The clinical features of focal epilepsy depend upon the site of the cortical focus. The two commoner types are:

1 **Temporal lobe (or complex partial) seizures**, which cause absences, olfactory hallucinations, *déja vu*, macropsia, automatisms such as lip smacking, or indescribable abdominal sensations.

2 **Focal motor convulsions**. An epileptic focus in the motor cortex, or adjacent frontal lobe, causes aversion of the head and eyes to the opposite side, or clonic contraction of the muscles of a hand, a foot, or one side of the face. These contractions may slowly 'march' to other parts of the body—**Jacksonian epilepsy**. Focal motor epileptic attacks may be followed by paralysis for a few hours of the limb(s) that had convulsed, **Todd's paralysis**. Phenytoin or carbamazepine are the most effective drugs for focal epilepsies.

Grand mal (or secondarily generalized) epilepsy

This is the commonest type of epilepsy in adults. Typically it involves tonic–clonic convulsions of the limbs, foaming at the mouth, postictal confusion, incontinence and tongue biting. In many patients it is

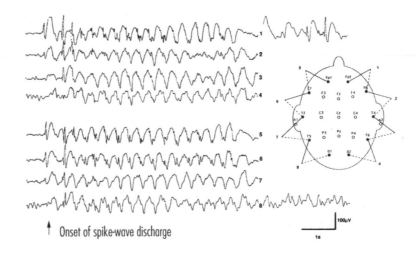

Fig. 21.2 An electroencephalogram (EEG) showing 3/sec spike and slow-wave discharge occurring in both cerebral hemispheres in a child with petit mal epilepsy.

↑ Onset of spike-wave discharge

100μV

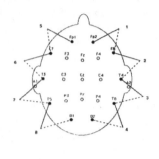

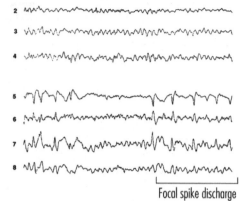

Focal spike discharge

Fig. 21.3 A focal seizure discharge in the left temporal lobe (leads 5, 6, and 7) in a patient with complex partial seizures (EEG).

due to rapid generalized spread of epileptic discharges throughout the brain from a focus (Fig. 21.4). For this reason it is essential to carry out **brain scans** in grand mal epilepsies principally to detect brain tumours. Modern high-resolution MRI is showing that 5–10 per cent have **cortical dysplasias**, which are focal anomalies of cerebral neuronal migration during development; often such epilepsies are intractable. An EEG is a much less valuable investigation in grand mal epilepsy than a brain scan.

Grand mal epilepsies usually respond to carbamazepine or phenytoin. Previously, phenobarbitone and primidone were the effective drugs, but have become unfashionable.

The single seizure

Patients who have had only one seizure are not regarded as suffering from the disease called epilepsy. However, a single seizure should be investigated with a brain scan to ensure that there is no underlying tumour. Patients with a single seizure are not usually treated with anticonvulsant drugs unless an underlying abnormality predisposing to further seizures is detected, such as a brain tumour.

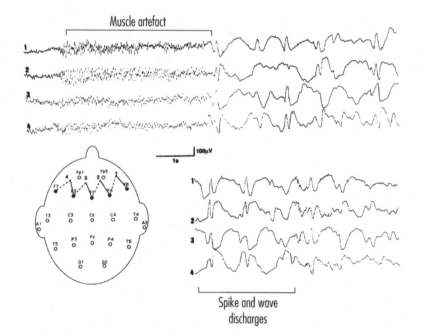

Spike and wave discharges

Fig. 21.4 A grand mal seizure discharge with irregular spikes and waves preceded by a few seconds of high-frequency muscle artefact as the convulsion began (EEG).

Status epilepticus

This is a sequence of seizures without full recovery of consciousness between. It can result in death, brain damage, or injury. The usual treatment is with respiratory support, controlling the seizures with intravenous benzodiazepines (such as diazepam), and loading with phenytoin. Intravenous barbiturate (thiopentone) is effective if diazepam fails.

Unfortunately a number of patients with recurrent psychogenic seizures (or **pseudoseizures**) are misdiagnosed as suffering from true status epilepticus. They get admitted to intensive care units where they risk iatrogenic injury as a result of well-meaning invasive procedures for therapy and monitoring. Pseudoseizures can be induced by suggestion and often show features uncommon in epilepsy, such as pelvic thrustings, resistance to eye opening, and prevention of a dropped hand from falling on the face. Cyanosis, tongue biting, and stereotyped attacks are uncommon. It is valuable to prove that seizure discharges are occurring by recording the EEG during status epilepticus.

Treatment of epilepsy

Anticonvulsant drugs

Four main drugs are used to treat epilepsy: carbamazepine, lamotrigine, phenytoin, and sodium valproate. A number of long-standing epileptics continue to take older but perfectly effective drugs such as phenobarbitone or primidone. Some useful new drugs have been introduced: clonazepam, gabapentin, topiramate, and vigabatrin. These newer drugs are generally used as add-on therapy in patients incompletely responsive to one of the main drugs. However, most patients with epilepsy can be treated satisfactorily with a single drug (monotherapy). Complicated drug interactions and side-effects may result from multiple therapy.

Mechanism of action

Most anticonvulsants seem to have multiple mechanisms of action at a cellular level. Almost all block repetitive neuronal firing by reducing neuronal sodium ion channel activity; phenytoin and carbamazepine are particular examples. Others augment γ-aminobutyric acid (GABA), the inhibitory neurotransmitter, for example sodium valproate, benzodiazepines, and barbiturates.

Carbamazepine

This is just as effective as phenytoin for treating grand mal and focal epilepsies. It replaced phenytoin because it does not have unwelcome cosmetic side-effects. Carbamazepine must be given twice or thrice daily.

Dangerous side-effects are rare but include sudden **agranulocytosis**, signalled by a sore throat, or **thrombocytopenia** causing a purpuric 'blood spot skin rash'. Patients should be warned to have a full blood count promptly in either event.

Lamotrigine

This recently introduced drug has a broad spectrum of activity against focal and generalized epilepsies. It is used as add-on therapy most often. Rash and acute hypersensitivity attacks are the main side-effects.

Phenytoin

This is highly effective for **grand mal** and **focal** epilepsies. It can be given once a day at night. Many patients develop side-effects of **facial hirsutes**, **coarsening of the skin**, **acne**, and **hypertrophied gums** which bleed.

Sodium valproate

This is the drug of choice for primarily generalized epilepsies such as childhood petit mal or juvenile myoclonic epilepsy. It is also effective in secondary generalized epilepsies. **Hepatic failure** is a rare complication; it has usually occurred in younger patients taking multiple anticonvulsant drugs. Mild **obesity** and thinning of the scalp hair are common side-effects. Polycystic ovarian syndrome can occur.

Monitoring anticonvulsant drug blood levels

This is not usually necessary when treating epileptics. Generally, drug doses should be adjusted so as to treat the patient's seizure disorder effectively, rather than to achieve a particular blood level. Levels are valuable for detecting **non-compliance**. Also, they can be useful to prove that the drug level is very high in patients with symptoms of **toxicity** such as mental dulling, vertigo, ataxia, and nystagmus. It can be informative to measure blood levels in patients receiving multiple drugs in whom metabolic interactions occur.

Anticonvulsant drugs in women of childbearing age

Three particular considerations govern the use of anticonvulsant drugs in women of childbearing age: **teratogenicity**, interaction with **oral contraceptives**, and **cosmetic** side-effects. Women with epilepsy should be alerted to the following points.

1 **Teratogenicity**. Epileptics have a three-fold increased risk of congenitally malformed babies. This risk is due partly to anticonvulsant drugs, and partly to the genetic load carried by the epileptic population. Carbamazepine is generally regarded as the safest drug

for women intending to become pregnant. Two drugs have been associated with particular malformations. **Phenytoin** is associated with craniofacial abnormalities such as cleft palate and also with congenital heart disease. **Sodium valproate** is associated with spina bifida. If sodium valproate is considered vital, or the pregnancy was inadvertent, the developing fetus should be monitored for neural tube defects by ultrasound scanning of the spine and α-fetoprotein measurement. The teratogenic potential of lamotrigine has not been determined and it is generally avoided in pregnancy. Regular **folic acid** administration should be given to women taking anticonvulsant drugs who intend to become pregnant so as to reduce the risk of neural tube defects.

2 **Oral contraception**. Phenytoin and carbamazepine increase the metabolism of oral contraceptive hormones leading to a 6- to 8-fold increase in the pill failure rate. This can be corrected by asking patients to take two, rather than one, oral contraceptive tablets daily. Sodium valproate and lamotrigine do not diminish the pill's contraceptive effectiveness.

3 **Cosmetic side-effects**. Phenytoin causes facial hirsutes, coarsening of the features, acne, and gum hypertrophy. Sodium valproate causes weight gain and thinning of the hair. Carbamazepine and lamotrigine are thankfully free of such cosmetic side-effects.

Thus carbamazepine is the anti-epileptic of choice in women. It is favoured in pregnancy on the grounds of lower teratogenicity and it is free of cosmetic side-effects. The oral contraceptive can still be used with carbamazepine as long as the pill dosage is increased.

Stopping anticonvulsant drugs

Overall, seizures recur in about a third of patients who have stopped their anticonvulsant drugs for 2 years. The risk of recurrence varies according to the type and severity of the epilepsy syndrome. For instance, by the time of adulthood, many childhood absence epilepsies have resolved. Many patients elect for long-term medication so as to avoid the risk of losing their driving licence if seizures recur. If anticonvulsants are to be stopped, it is best to reduce the dosage progressively over a few months.

Driving regulations

The UK driving and vehicle licensing authority (DVLA) has statutory restrictions for epileptics. Similar regulations apply after single seizures and for those with other unpredictable blackouts which could impair driving. Any patient with a single seizure, or a diagnosis of epilepsy (two or more seizures) is obliged to stop driving until they have been free of attacks for 1 year. This applies whether they are taking anticonvulsant drugs or not. This restriction includes those with more minor epileptic disturbances, such as complex partial seizures. It is the patient's obligation to inform the DVLA themselves. The doctor would be breaking confidentially if he reported the patient directly, and should merely remind the patient of their own obligation to inform the DVLA. Driving bans pose major obstacles to employment and family life. On hearing of the prospect of a ban some patients deliberately fail to tell the DVLA and continue driving. Others may question the diagnosis somewhat angrily and sometimes seek a second opinion when, interestingly, they may give a different history.

Vasovagal attacks (simple faints)

Most people have either fainted, or had a threatened faint, at some time in their lives. Faints usually occur when standing up. The postural hypotension reduces brain perfusion, which leads to unconsciousness. Prompt recovery occurs once the patient has fallen horizontally. Whilst unconscious, the patient lies **motionless**.

Attacks are precipitated particularly by diversion of blood to the portal circulation by heavy meals, or to vasodilated hot skin after a hot bath, by hangovers and tiredness, by pain or the sight of blood or other stomach churning experiences, or by standing micturating. Carotid sinus syncope can result from tight collars.

Patients can usually remember feeling as though their consciousness was draining away. This 'draining away' often involves unsteadiness, vertigo, or blacking out of vision. As soon as they regain consciousness patients are well oriented, with a clear memory of the onset.

Occasionally **reflex anoxic seizures** occur if a fainting patient is held upright and prevented from falling, thus suffering more prolonged cerebral ischaemia.

Cardiac blackouts

Complete heart block, or tachyarrhythmias with poor cerebral perfusion, may cause a **Stokes–Adams attack**. The patient becomes completely unconsciousness over a few seconds, and becomes deathly **pale**. The diagnosis is proven if a competent witness has failed to detect the pulse. If a good cardiac output returns before significant cerebral anoxia has occurred, the patient wakes up properly and is well oriented with a clear memory of the onset. It is often difficult to prove retrospectively that a blackout was due to a cardiac arrhythmia. Twenty-four hour electrocardiograph monitoring may show that a patient is having arrhythmias, although it rarely catches an arrhythmic episode that proves the diagnosis beyond doubt.

Hyperventilation attacks

Some anxious individuals have attacks of breathing excessively thereby blowing off carbon dioxide and causing a **respiratory alkalosis**. This reduces the ionized calcium level in the blood. These patients are often unaware of breathing excessively. They may be aware of having 'difficulty in filling my chest with air' at the onset, or feelings of non-specific giddiness. Tinglings in the fingers and around the mouth, or spasms of the small hand muscles are typical. They are due to spontaneous discharges in hyperexcitable nerves caused by hypocalcaemia. Such patients often dip in and out of semiconsciousness for half an hour or so without ever having a clearly defined period of complete and profound unconsciousness. Epileptic convulsions rarely occur, although tremulous movements of the fingers may be observed and misinterpreted as true convulsions. Hyperventilation attacks can be terminated promptly by **rebreathing** from a paper bag. This reverses the respiratory alkalosis and restores the ionized calcium level in the blood to normal. You can precipitate an attack in the clinic by asking the patient to hyperventilate voluntarily, and then terminating the attack by rebreathing. This is a valuable diagnostic test and it provides the patient with an instructive insight.

Hypoglycaemic attacks

These are rare. Low blood glucose occurs in adults with depleted liver glycogen reserves following alcoholic binges or starvation, in insulin-secreting pancreatic islet cell tumours, or after overdosage with hypoglycaemic drugs such as insulin. The chief features are hunger, sweating, nervousness, and palpitations, progressing to **coma**. Hyperglycaemic convulsions may occur. It is difficult to prove the diagnosis because the blood sugar is rarely measured during the height of an attack. Prolonged hypoglycaemia causes permanent brain damage. Thus, when faced with an undiagnosed unconscious patient, you should give intravenous glucose whilst you await the result of blood tests and brain scans.

CASE 21.1 'AN EVOLVING STORY'

An office executive of 60 was referred because of temporary loss of memory a few weeks previously. This had lasted 3 or 4 hours, spanning lunchtime and the early afternoon. Subsequently, he had been able to deduce from the empty wrapper on his desk and the change in his pocket that he had been to the canteen and bought a sandwich, apparently behaving normally. Two colleagues said that he had held sensible telephone conversations with them, of which he had no subsequent memory. A diagnosis of transient global amnesia was made, and he was reassured that more than occasional occurrences were unusual. A few months later he was re-referred because of three more such attacks. One had lasted only 20 minutes, which is unusually short for transient global amnesia. In another, a work colleague had found him to be confused about the purpose of a document he himself had drafted. A brain scan and an EEG were normal. No definitive diagnosis could be made, but he was given a follow-up appointment for re-evaluation because the story was becoming atypical for the original diagnosis. Just a few weeks later he had a grand mal seizure. He was given carbamazepine on the hypothesis that his amnesic attacks had been an unusual form of complex partial seizure. No more amnesic attacks occurred.

Comment

◆ Transient global amnesia is a phenomenon affecting middle-aged or elderly patients who complain of having no memory of events for a few hours. Despite this, eye witnesses usually report that they were behaving both rationally and normally. There may be evidence that they drove a sensible route, or undertook some necessary shopping.

◆ Often only a single attack of transient global amnesia ever occurs. More than a handful of attacks is unusual. It is a rather distinctive and fascinating syndrome whose cause is not known, although thalamic transient ischaemic attacks or migraine equivalents (i.e. without headache) have been hypothesized.

◆ Although this patient's first attack seemed typical of transient global amnesia, the subsequent history showed that his amnesic attacks had an epileptic basis. The clues to this were the short duration and relative frequency of the attacks, and ultimately the occurrence of a secondarily generalized seizure.

CHAPTER 22

Sleepiness and coma

Daytime sleepiness

It is hard to define when daytime sleepiness is excessive and therefore pathological. It is obviously abnormal if someone falls asleep during meals or demanding tasks. But many normal adolescents and young adults need lots of sleep, as any lecturer knows. Excessive sleepiness is socially embarrassing. It can cause accidents if it occurs whilst driving or working with machinery. The two most important disorders are the narcolepsy–cataplexy syndrome and obstructive sleep apnoea. Hypothalamic tumours are an occasional cause of somnolence.

The narcolepsy–cataplexy syndrome

Narcoleptic patients cannot stop themselves falling asleep despite having had a good night's sleep. They may have **cataplexy** in which laughter or anger make their muscles temporarily weak, sometimes so that they have to sit down. They can describe frightening episodes of **sleep paralysis** in bed in which they cannot move a muscle voluntarily but continue breathing. **Hypnagogic hallucinations** may occur in the twilight zone whilst falling asleep. These often have a strongly visual nature with abstract shapes and vivid colours. **Sleep myoclonus** may occur excessively; although most of us have occasional attacks of myoclonic jerking associated with an illusion of falling at the time of falling asleep.

Narcolepsy normally starts in the late teens or early twenties. The diagnosis depends principally upon a clear history of excessive daytime sleepiness and cataplexy. Typically such patients enter directly into the rapid eye movement (REM) phase of sleep if the EEG is recorded whilst they fall asleep. The **HLA DR2 antigen** is almost invariably present, which implies a genetic susceptibility. If narcolepsy is disabling or potentially dangerous, it can be treated with amphetamines, methylphenidate, or modafinil. Cataplexy can be abolished with tricyclic drugs such as clomipramine.

Obstructive sleep apnoea

These patients fall asleep during the day because they have not obtained a restful and refreshing night's sleep due to obstructed breathing. Their sleeping companion will describe loud **snoring**, with frequent **apnoeic episodes** lasting 30 seconds or so in which the patient frantically tries to breathe through a blocked throat. Strangulated **choking** noises occur during these episodes. During the apnoeic attacks the patient often struggles and kicks off the bedclothes, before starting to breathe freely again. The cumulative effects of these apnoeic attacks deprive the patient of refreshing and prolonged deep sleep.

The apnoea results from mechanical obstruction in the pharynx due to a fat neck, large tonsils, or a large tongue. In addition, poor muscle tone in the upper respiratory tract may promote **pharyngal collapse** during inspiration. Unlike narcolepsy, sleepiness due to obstructive sleep apnoea tends to start in middle age. Obstructive sleep apnoea is associated with an increased risk of sudden cardio-respiratory death. The diagnosis can be proved by observing and monitoring respiratory movements and blood oxygen saturation during sleep. Treatments include losing weight, tonsillectomy, and sleeping wearing a face mask which delivers positive airway pressure.

Occasionally sleep apnoea is due to brainstem lesions affecting the respiratory centres, usually due to infarction. This causes arrest of breathing movements rather than airway obstruction.

Coma

A patient in **coma** appears to be asleep but is completely unrousable. **Stupor** is a halfway state between coma and consciousness in which patients can be roused by intense stimulation, but remain sleepy, slow, and inattentive. Stupor and coma generally have the same causes. The individual causes are unmemorably numerous. Thus it is useful to remember the categories given in Table 22.1.

Diagnosis

The diagnosis is often obvious from the circumstances: for instance, an alcoholic binge, a head injury, a cardiac arrest, diabetes, or a seizure without resumption of

TABLE 22.1 Seven types of coma
Poisonings (drugs, alcohol)
Head injury (concussion, subdural haematoma, extradural haematoma)
Stroke (subarachnoid haemorrhage, large cerebral infarcts or haematomas)
Status epilepticus (convulsive or non-convulsive)
Metabolic (diabetic, uraemic, hepatic)
Infective (meningitis, encephalitis)
Anoxic (pneumonia, hypoxic–hypotensive encephalopathy)

consciousness. If there is no such clue to the cause, the cardiorespiratory and neurological systems must be examined carefully, and blood taken for glucose, creatinine, and toxicological analysis. Cardiovascular examination may reveal shock or arrhythmia. Neurological examination may reveal:

- neck stiffness (meningitis, subarachnoid haemorrhage);
- generalized or focal seizures (status epilepticus, encephalitis);
- brainstem damage (pin-point pupils, loss of the vestibulo-ocular, corneal, or gag reflexes);
- hemiparesis (failure to withdraw one side to pain) (stroke, trauma, encephalitis);
- papilloedema (raised intracranial pressure).

If any of these neurological findings are present an urgent brain scan is necessary, followed by spinal fluid examination if it is normal. If acute meningitis is suspected, blood should be cultured and penicillin treatment given before the brain scan. Patients in coma often require assisted ventilation and circulatory support, whilst you await the results of diagnostic tests or wait for specific treatments to start working.

Brain death

Some causes of coma lead to irrecoverable brain damage. Most usually this follows head injury, subarachnoid haemorrhage, cerebral infarction, intracerebral haematoma, untreated meningitis, or hypoxic–hypotensive encephalopathy due to prolonged cardiac arrest. Once brain death is diagnosed according to specified criteria, ventilation can be discontinued and the patient's internal organs considered for transplant donation. To declare a patient brain dead you must be satisfied that there is:

1 no reversible and recoverable disorder;

2 no loss of brainstem reflexes such as caloric eye movements or pupil responses;

3 failure of the patient's unaided respiration to maintain blood oxygenation.

You must also be sure that the patient is truly comatose and not merely '**locked in**'—in other words fully conscious and able to see but unable to hear, feel, or move because of brainstem damage. Locked-in patients can often move their eyes to stimuli, and move their eyes voluntarily if only upwards.

Persistent vegetative state

Modern intensive care allows many patients to survive from coma. A proportion of these develop a **persistent vegetative state** in which they self-ventilate and open their eyes spontaneously. But they display no evidence of awareness or purposeful activity and can only be kept alive by skilled nursing, including nasogastric feeding. The extent to which such patients should be kept alive is a matter of considerable ethical and legal debate.

CASE 22.1 'SLEEPING POLICEMAN'

After apprehension, some local villains were nonplussed to find the burly duty gendarme falling asleep whilst booking them into the cells. Narcolepsy had been entertained as the diagnosis to explain his excessive daytime sleepiness. However, he did not have other elements of that syndrome, such as cataleptic sagging of his body musculature during emotions, episodes of sleep paralysis, or sleep myoclonus. Whilst quietly contemplating possible diagnoses it became evident that his breathing was extremely noisy. Madame had noted that his breathing often obstructed for short periods whilst asleep, during which he would struggle and disrupt their bedclothes. He had snored heavily for years and this had worsened. Recently his collar size had increased due to neck obesity. The suspected diagnosis of obstructive sleep apnoea was confirmed by sleep recordings which showed episodes of blocked airflow in his upper airways despite continued respiratory effort. Dips in the oxygen saturation of the blood occurred simultaneously. For sleeping he was fitted with a continuous positive airways pressure system delivered via a facial mask. He managed to lose some weight and an otorhinolaryngologist trimmed away chronically enlarged tonsils which were contributing to his obstruction. With the resultant improvement in the quality of his sleep, his daytime sleepiness resolved.

Comment

♦ Narcolepsy and obstructive sleep apnoea are the common causes to consider for excessive daytime sleepiness.

♦ Obstructive sleep apnoea produces mild hypoxaemia. Also it diminishes the amount of time patients spend in those deeper stages of sleep which are necessary for dreaming and proper rest.

♦ Chronic daytime sleepiness is a serious condition which increases the risk of road traffic accidents due to falling asleep at the wheel.

♦ Asking the patient's spouse about snoring and episodes of obstruction whilst asleep is a crucial clue to the diagnosis of obstructive sleep apnoea.

Speech disorders

Speech disturbances

There are three types of speech disturbance:

1 **dysphonia**: inability to make noise properly with the larynx;

2 **dysarthria**: inability to shape that noise accurately into recognizable sounds;

3 **dysphasia**: difficulty with understanding or formulating language.

Dysphonia

Dysphonia is due either to paralysis of the vocal cords or to structural disease of the larynx such as laryngitis or tumours. **Vocal cord paralysis** produces quiet speech punctuated by frequent breaths because so much air is required to make any noise. You can prove that a vocal cord is paralysed by asking the patient to give a sharp cough. Instead of the normal explosive cough produced by sudden opening of the larynx, a paralysed larynx causes a cough which is 'bovine' – having a gradual onset and a bellowing quality. Vocal cord paralysis can arise from motor neuron disease affecting the vagus motor neurons, from myasthenic weakness of laryngeal muscles, from polyneuropathy such as Guillain–Barré syndrome affecting laryngeal nerves, or from focal mononeuropathy of a laryngeal nerve. Focal lesions usually affect the long recurrent laryngeal nerve on the left. Typical causes include compression by bronchial carcinoma or aortic arch aneurism as the nerve loops under the aortic arch.

Dysarthria

Dysarthria is due to an inability to coordinate the tongue, pharynx, and lip muscles so as to form consonants. It is best tested by words with lots of consonants such as 'uNiVeRSiTy', 'WeST ReGiSTeR STReeT', or 'BRiTiSH CoNSTiTuTioN'. Try saying the following consonants: 'G, T, P, K, S, L', whilst noting what is going on inside your mouth. You will realize that each depends on a specific configuration and movement profile of the tongue, palate, and lips. Cerebellar incoordination will make these consonants slurred and slow; thus many people with multiple sclerosis have a scanning dysarthria. A pseudobulbar palsy produces a spastic immobile tongue which cannot form consonants and leads to 'hot potato speech' or even total anarthria (absence of speech).

Dysphasia

Dysphasia results from damage to the speech areas of the left cerebral hemisphere. This lateralization holds in all except a minority of left-handed people. Once you detect dysphasia, you should arrange a brain scan; the commonest causes are tumours and infarcts. Temporary dysphasia may occur with classical migraine, embolic transient ischaemic attacks, or focal epilepsies. When assessing dysphasic speech you should listen to a free flow of speech as the patient describes some aspect of their everyday life.

There are two main types of dysphasia: **receptive** and **motor**. Note whether the patient's speech is **fluent** (words are produced at the normal rate) or **non-fluent** (long pauses due to word-finding difficulty). Also note whether the speech is **jumbled up** and meaningless, or whether wrong words occur. Can the patient understand a verbal command?

Receptive, sensory, or Wernicke's dysphasia

Although the speech is **fluent**, it is meaningless because the words are wrong or jumbled up. The patient cannot understand a simple three or four component command such as 'when I clap my hands, but not before, could you touch your left ear with your right index finger'. The patient cannot read instructions either. Receptive dysphasia results from lesions at the junction between the left temporal and parietal lobes (Wernicke's area; Fig. 23.1).

Motor or Broca's aphasia

The speech is **non-fluent** with great gaps devoid of words. Sometimes the patient cannot utter at all even though they can move their tongue properly. Habitual expressions such as 'Good morning' or 'Thank you' may be preserved, but the rest of speech is halting and expressionless. The patient is aware that their speech is defective and may grimace to express their frustration,

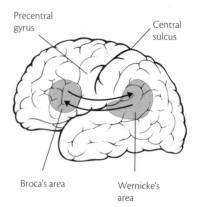

Fig. 23.1 Broca's and Wernicke's areas. Diagrammatic view of the surface of the left cerebral hemisphere.

or use gestures to try and add meaning to their attempts at speech. Broca's aphasia results from a lesion at the bottom of the precentral gyrus (Fig. 23.1). If the lesion is large, and extends into the adjacent motor cortex it may also cause weakness of the right side of the face.

Global aphasia

Large lesions that involve both Broca's and Wernicke's areas cause global aphasia, which is a combined motor and sensory dysphasia. Very mild dysphasias of either type can be detected best by the ability to name items such as body parts, items of clothing, or parts of a watch.

Distinguishing aphasia from dementia

Language is our normal window to the functions of the rest of cognition. Not surprisingly it can be difficult to distinguish between a pure aphasia and the disturbed language that is part of a generalized dementia. However, demented patients will not use non-verbal communication normally, whereas aphasic patients consciously overemphasize smiles or gestures to compensate for their poor speech. Nurses and relatives note that demented patients fail to learn simple spatial tasks, such as the location of the ward lavatory. The disturbed spatial function due to right parietal lobe abnormalities in dementia may cause a dressing apraxia which can be tested without speech. Dressing apraxia renders a patient unable to put on a garment, such as a dressing gown, with one sleeve pulled inside out.

CHAPTER 24

Neuropsychological syndromes and dementia

Neuropsychological syndromes

Certain clusters of neuropsychological deficits characterize damage to particular areas of the cerebral hemispheres. Information about these syndromes comes from studying patients with strokes, tumours, or brain trauma, particularly from gunshot wounds.

The frontal lobes

These are most highly developed in primates, particularly humans. Yet their function has proved remarkably difficult to define. On superficial assessment, the clinical effects of anatomically substantial lesions can appear rather mild. Frontal damage changes the personality. Most usually patients become **disinhibited** with childish excitement, joking, indiscretions of sexual and excretory behaviour, and exhibitionism. In others, the frontal lobe syndrome is predominantly a lack of initiative and concern with loss of social awareness for excretory functions. The patient may become unkempt, lack spontaneity, and manifest primitive reflexes such as sucking and rooting. It is the spouse who usually notices the milder behavioural change of an early frontal lobe lesion, feeling that 'he is not the man I married'. Sometimes one has noted that slow-growing tumours of the frontal lobe have become clinically evident only in the aftermath of marital breakdown.

If the deeper and more posterior structures of the frontal lobe are affected, **gait apraxia** occurs (see Chapter 25). Also, patients may find it impossible to

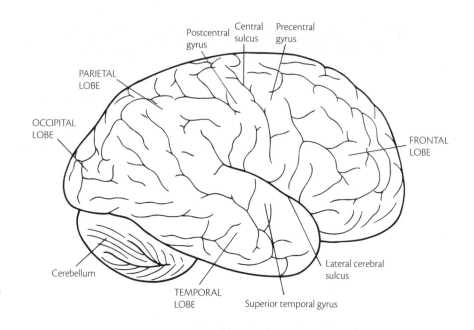

Fig. 24.1 Lateral view of the lobes of the brain.

relax the tone when their legs are being examined, so-called **gegenhalten**. Doctors often regard this as an irritating obstacle to examination without realizing its diagnostic significance. Posteriorly located lesions in the dominant (left) frontal lobe produce a non-fluent motor or Broca-type dysphasia (see Chapter 23).

The temporal lobes

Bilateral temporal lobe lesions can produce a distressing change in behaviour. Such lesions occur after herpes encephalitis or the type of fronto-temporal degeneration which used to be known as Pick's disease. Involvement of the dominant temporal lobe produces sensory or **Wernicke-type dysphasia** (see Chapter 23). Bilateral disruption of the hippocampus and other structures of the limbic system leads to profound **memory disturbance**, particularly for recent events. Hypersexuality, obsessional behaviour, altered eating habits, or hyper-religiosity may occur. In some patients the personality and behaviour are so profoundly disturbed that they react to any stimulus by excessive **rage**, with screaming and biting.

A unilateral lesion affecting a single temporal lobe does not impair memory or behaviour. Apart from dysphasia, when lesions affect the dominant temporal lobe, the main features are visual. Involvement of the lower fibres of the optic radiation produces a superior quadrantic homonymous **visual field defect**. Disturbances of visual and auditory perception also occur, particularly with lesions of the non-dominant temporo-parietal areas. **Prosopagnosia** is an inability to recognize faces. **Amusia** is loss of the ability to appreciate and recognize music.

The parietal lobes

The parietal lobes are enormous, and a considerable range of neuropsychological deficits can follow damage.

Dominant parietal lobe lesions are associated with **dysphasia**. **Dyslexia** (difficulty with reading), **dysgraphia** (difficulty with writing), **dyscalculia** (impaired arithmetic ability), and **right–left disorientation** occur. **Apraxia** is an inability to carry out a complex motor function despite normal motor power. When asked, the patient may be unable to voluntarily protrude their tongue, despite later protruding it spontaneously to lick their lips.

Damage to the non-dominant (right) parietal lobe causes striking disturbances of spatial orientation and body image. The left side of the body may be totally neglected with the jacket sleeve hanging empty and that side of the face unshaven. In milder lesions, simultaneous presentation of touch or visual stimuli to the two sides of the body results in **inattention** contralateral to the parietal lobe lesion. **Astereognosis** is an inability to recognize objects by their shape, such as coins in a pocket. Patients may leave out features from the left side when asked to draw a clock face or have no concept of their clothes as three-dimensional objects. Such **dressing apraxia** is best tested by asking a patient to put on a jacket with one sleeve pulled through the wrong way.

The occipital lobes

The occipital lobes are entirely devoted to vision. Damage to the primary visual cortex in the occipital pole produces homonymous hemianopia in the contralateral field (see Chapter 14). Extensive bilateral lesions can cause complete cortical blindness, in which the pupil–light response is preserved. More anterior lesions of the occipital lobes can produce selective loss of colour or movement perception, or **visual agnosias**, which are inabilities to recognize objects by sight.

Dementia

Dementia is a generalized loss of cognitive function, including memory, due to diffuse disease of both cerebral hemispheres. To begin with, the symptoms are minor and may be attributed to absent mindedness. Then **errors of judgement** are noted, and the ability to perform a familiar intellectual task such as crosswords deteriorates. Alarm is generated eventually by failure to remember the grandchildren's names and by loss of interest in long-standing hobbies and recreations.

Later the personality is lost; 'he is not the same man as I married'. Gross loss of memory and judgement become evident, and the patient starts getting lost in familiar places. Sometimes demented patients become untalkative. Others may become distressingly repetitive or perseverative. Frontal lobe involvement causes **disinhibition** about the normal social rules governing excretory and sexual behaviour. Eventually the patient is mute and unresponsive, wanders aimlessly, is incontinent, and has to be fed, ultimately becoming bedridden and dying of bronchopneumonia.

Diagnosing advanced dementia is not difficult, but diagnosing early dementia can be. The basic neurological examination is usually normal. The patient is rather uninformative, vague, or rambling during history taking. Cognitive examination reveals dyscalculia in which the 100-7 test is performed slowly and inaccurately, or is impossible. Amnesia for recent events is shown by inability to remember a simple three-line name and address even after practice. The patient may be dysphasic. Apraxia is shown by the inability to use common everyday implements even though there is no elementary motor disorder affecting the hands. Disorientation for date, place, and person occurs. Cognitive estimates provide a simple test of judgment; questions such as 'How many camels are there in Holland?' are answered inaccurately. Spatial disorientation due to right parietal lobe involvement is shown by an inability to draw a cube in three dimensions, or by dressing apraxia. General knowledge is poor. The patient has little or no insight into these difficulties. There is obvious neglect of social graces, codes of behaviour, and personal appearance.

Causes

Usually dementia is due to incurable disorders such as **Alzheimer's disease** or **multiple cerebral infarctions**. Although rare, Creutzfeldt–Jakob disease (Chapter 28) causes rapidly deteriorating dementia. An important aim of investigation is to uncover potentially reversible or stoppable causes:

1 Brain scan will show **hydrocephalus** requiring shunting, or rare abnormalities such as **frontal tumours**.

2 **Metabolic and infective disorders** (vitamin B_{12} deficiency, hypercalcaemia, thyroid deficiency, syphilis, HIV infection).

3 **Toxic causes** such as chronic alcoholism or chronic barbiturate consumption.

4 **Pseudo-dementia** due to depression may be treated with antidepressants. Apart from their symptoms of depression, such patients usually show an unusual degree of concern and insight about their memory loss.

Multi-infarct dementia

Vascular dementia is common and may coexist with Alzheimer's disease. It is due to multiple cerebral infarcts in each cerebral hemisphere, often predominantly in the sub-cortical white matter. These infarcts are evident on MRI or CT scanning. There are two main differences from Alzheimer's disease. First, multi-infarct dementia progresses in a **step-wise manner** rather than deteriorating progressively. Secondly, physical signs of **focal damage**, such as visual field defects, focal weakness, or an extensive plantar response, are more likely. Investigation aims to detect removable sources of cerebral emboli. Treatment includes aspirin prophylaxis and controlling hypertension.

Normal pressure hydrocephalus

This potentially treatable form of **dementia** is suggested by the associated urinary **incontinence** and **gait apraxia**. Gait apraxia is an exaggerated form of the short-stepping gait familiar in old people. Brain scans show distended cerebral ventricles. Normal pressure hydrocephalus is due to a disorder of cerebral–spinal fluid flow, with intermittent waves of high pressure, although routine measurement of CSF pressure by lumbar puncture is normal. Once suspected, the patient should be admitted to hospital for lumbar puncture drainage of spinal fluid on three consecutive days to see if walking speed, mental test scores, and incontinence improve. If so, valuable long-term improvement may be achieved by permanent CSF drainage via a ventriculo-peritoneal shunt.

Alzheimer's disease

Alzheimer's disease poses a huge social and medical problem, which is steadily increasing as the population becomes older. Many long-stay psychiatric patients have Alzheimer's disease, and the disease causes incalculable disruption and distress within families. It is rare before the age of 50 but gets commoner thereafter. Alzheimer's disease involves loss of neurons from the cerebral cortex and hippocampus associated with characteristic plaques of deposited amyloid and neurofibrillary tangles. MR scans are normal in the early stages of Alzheimer's disease, but show generalized brain atrophy later, which particularly affects the hippocampus, thus explaining the prominent memory deficits.

Alzheimer's disease follows the clinical course of dementia described above. Memory loss is particularly prominent early on, but general loss of cognitive abilities becomes evident as the years pass. Alzheimer's disease usually continues to deteriorate for at least 5 years. Centrally acting cholinesterase-inhibiting drugs can produce mild, although useful, improvement in the neuropsychological disturbances of mild to moderate Alzheimer's disease. These drugs boost the low levels of brain acetylcholine that result from loss of choline acetyltransferase-containing neurons in Alzheimer's disease, which may underlie the amnesia.

Causes

Most Alzheimer's disease is sporadic, and the abnormality of neuronal biology has not been identified. A central feature is the deposition of β-amyloid protein within plaques in the cerebral cortex. One of the three alleles (E4) of the apolipoprotein E gene confers susceptibility for developing Alzheimer's disease in the general population. A few patients have autosomal dominant familial Alzheimer's disease. This can involve mutations of the amyloid precursor protein gene, or other genes (presenilin) that affect the metabolism of this precursor protein.

Other neurodegenerative dementia syndromes

Frontotemporal degenerations involve focal atrophy of these lobes of the cerebral cortex, with the associated behavioural and neuropsychological disturbances. They include the sporadic disorder known as Pick's disease, and autosomal dominant disorders caused by mutations in the gene encoding Tau. Tau is a protein associated with microtubules, and other Tau gene mutations can cause dementia syndromes characterized by **supranuclear gaze palsy**, in which voluntary gaze is impaired, and **corticobasal degeneration**, in which a hand may move with a mind of its own. **Dementia with Lewy bodies** is associated with mutations of the α-synuclein gene; there is associated Parkinson's disease, and prominent confusion and hallucinations. Not all **Creutzfeldt–Jakob** disease occurs sporadically; autosomal dominant transmission of prion protein gene mutations can produce this rapidly progressive dementia associated with myoclonic jerkings.

CASE 24.1 'I'M A FRIEND OF THE KING'

A man in his 50s required intravenous feeding for some weeks after extensive upper gastrointestinal tract surgery. He was a rather malnourished man, who drank heavily, lived alone, and whose employment as an odd-job man contrasted with his educational and social background. The neurologists were asked to see him because he became unrousable over a couple of days. When examining this stuporous man on the intensive care unit, the most striking feature was the complete loss of gaze movements to shouting or hand waving, and a loss of reflex eye movements when his head was turned. His ankle jerks were absent. Intravenous injection of thiamine (vitamin B_1) produced a striking improvement in conscious level and eye movements over the next 8 hours. Indeed, these features changed strikingly from hour to hour during the night. Water-soluble vitamins had not been included in the parenteral feeding regimen until that point.

The patient was seen a couple of months later following recovery from his surgery and discharge from hospital. Initially all seemed well, although his reply about the current monarch of 'King George' was some decades out of date. When asked if he was sure it was King George, he replied that he had met him just last week, and had found him to be well. It transpired that he was unable to remember his recent stay in hospital. It was never discovered how he had managed to keep his outpatient appointment.

Comment

- This patient had acute Wernicke's encephalopathy. The typical features are somnolence and complex eye movement disorders.

- Wernicke's encephalopathy is due to thiamine (vitamin B_1) deficiency. Normally the bodily supplies will last 6–8 weeks, but they were clearly reduced in this malnourished patient with a history of alcoholism. The disorder was precipitated by a high-calorific intravenous feeding regimen devoid of thiamine for only 2 weeks.

- Administration of intravenous thiamine is required urgently when Wernicke's encephalopathy is suspected. If the diagnosis is correct, the clinical response can be so striking that it is one of the few phenomena in medicine which is worth staying out of bed to observe.

- Later this man was noted to have a residual disorder of recent memory of the type known as Korsakoff's syndrome. In this, patients cannot lay down recent memories, although they can remember the past, and often confabulate to fill in the gaps with seemingly plausible explanations.

- Vitamin B_1 deficiency is not the only cause of a Korsakoff syndrome. It can also be due to any cause of bilateral damage to the limbic system, such as infarcts of the dorsomedial thalamus or bilateral temporal lobe damage due to herpes encephalitis.

- In alcoholics, features of mild Wernicke encephalopathy and the Korsakoff amnesic syndrome often coexist. For this reason, the complex is often referred to as the 'Wernicke–Korsakoff syndrome'.

- Vitamin B_1 deficiency can affect the peripheral nervous system too; indeed this patient's ankle jerks were absent and he had sensory ataxia due to proprioceptive loss from the legs. This is the syndrome of dry beri-beri, as opposed to wet beri-beri in which oedema occurs due to heart failure.

- Thiamine deficiency is not the main cause of dementia in alcoholics. So-called 'alcoholic dementia' usually reflects varying combinations of acute intoxication, mild delirium tremens, depression, focal cerebral trauma due to falls, subdural haematoma, and diffuse alcohol toxicity to the brain.

CHAPTER 25

Gait disorders and falls

Analysing gait

Walking is a complex motor performance which naturally changes with age. Everyone's gait has its own characteristics—one can normally recognize an acquaintance by their walk even when too far away to recognize their face. The range of disease that affects walking is enormous. Non-neurological disorders, such as hip joint disease, are common. In the elderly, gait disorders may have multiple causes, for instance, a combination of Parkinsonism, hip joint arthritis, and the mild apraxia of natural ageing.

Normal gait

It is important to understand normal gait, and to analyse its abnormalities, so as to recognize the abnormal characteristics associated with various diseases.

Separation of the feet

Normally the feet cross within a few centimetres of each other during a stride, leading to occasional scuffs on the inner heel of shoes. In a normally efficient gait, the feet touch the ground almost in a straight line, and loop slightly round each other during striding (Fig. 25.1(a)). Wide-based gait occurs in ataxia due to cerebellar disease or loss of proprioceptive feedback. A slightly wide-based gait can also occur in apraxia or Parkinson's disease, but is associated with a short stride length in both these conditions. The feet cross in wide arcs in spastic gaits because the stiffly extended leg and foot cannot be flexed in the normal manner so as to clear the ground during a stride.

Stride length

Normally one hits a standard length stride with the first step and it varies little thereafter. The stride length is variable in ataxia with elongated strides leading to overbalancing and shortened strides causing stumbling over a foot that has gone down too soon (Fig. 25.1(b)). Shortened, shuffling strides occur in Parkinson's disease. The gait ignition failure of more advanced Parkinson's disease leads to a hesitant start to a walk and

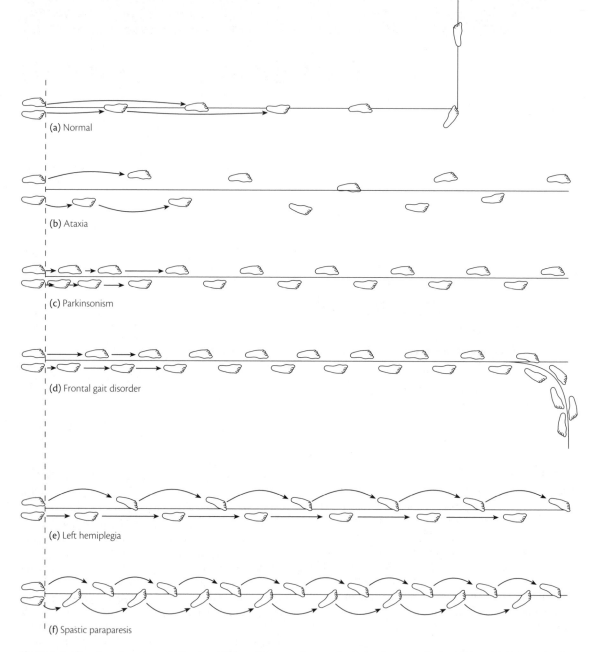

Fig. 25.1 Stride patterns in various gait disorders. (a) The stride pattern in normal gait showing how a fixed stride length is hit immediately, and varies little thereafter, how the feet cross close to one another, and how a corner is taken in a single step by spinning on the foot through a right angle. (b) Ataxia showing wide separation of the feet and an irregular stride length. (c) Parkinsonism showing short strides, with a shuffling start. (d) Frontal gait disorder, gait apraxia, or *marche à petits pas*, showing the short steps and walking round corners, rather than spinning round them. (e) and (f) Showing a left hemiplegia and spastic paraparesis, respectively, with circumduction of the spastic leg(s).

acceleration associated with increasing stride length (Fig. 25.1(c)). Gait apraxias, or frontal gait disorders, cause short striding of constant length from the start, a so-called *marche à petits pas* (Fig. 25.1(d)). In its milder forms this looks like a typical old person's gait. Apraxic patients have particular difficulty in turning corners, being unable to turn round at a single step, and sometimes getting their feet hopelessly tangled up and having to walk in a wide circle around corners (Fig. 25.1(d)).

Foot drop

Foot drop prevents the patient from swinging their striding leg through underneath their body without catching it on the ground. This causes them to trip over their toe, and shows itself as wearing out of the toe of their shoe. There are two types of foot drop gaits: stiffly held and floppy.

Stiff foot drop usually results from spasticity, and less frequently from dystonia. Walking with a spastic leg requires laborious circumduction of the stiffly extended leg and foot in a wide lateral arc so as to avoid catching the toe (Fig. 25.1(e)). This compensatory manoeuvre is required bilaterally in spastic paraparesis (Fig. 25.1(f)). Such scissors gait is exhaustingly inefficient, and throws unnatural stresses on the low back and pelvic girdle, which can result in further gait deterioration due to secondary degenerative arthritis. Occasionally stiff foot drop is due to dystonia, in which case the plantar response is not extensor.

Floppy foot drops occur with lower motor neuron weakness of tibialis anterior. This is unilateral in L5/S1 root lesions, or common peroneal nerve lesions. It is bilateral in polyneuropathy or motor neuron diseases. In order to swing the dangling foot through during a stride without catching it on the ground, the hip and knee are flexed exaggeratedly so as to lift the leg, and the foot is kicked out in front to land on the ground. A good example is the gait of the television detective, Inspector Morse.

Waddling gait

Normally the pelvis stays level during walking due to contraction of gluteus medius on the weight-bearing side during a stride. If there is proximal muscle weakness due to myopathy, the pelvis flops down towards the side on which the leg is lifted from the ground to take a stride. This gives the gait a waddling appearance.

Arm swing

Normally balance is assisted by swinging the arm opposite to the striding leg, familiar in its most exaggerated form in military marching. Loss of arm swing is charac-

teristic of Parkinson's disease, occurring unilaterally in the early stages. Arm swing of irregular amplitude, sometimes of a slightly wild nature, may occur in ataxia, in part as a balance compensatory mechanism.

Rising and standing

Rising and standing depend upon righting reflexes and supporting reflexes, respectively. Some patients with high-level gait disorders can be unable to make it into the upright position, or to maintain their centre of gravity over their feet when there. Other patients may lose postural adjustment responses to unexpected displacements, or spontaneous imbalances or trips.

Types of gait disorder

It is useful to consider a hierarchy of gait disorder types. Patients are well able to compensate and continue walking with low-level gait disorders, whereas they often lose the ability to walk at all with high-level disorders.

Low-level gait disorders

These usually result from disorders of the skeleton, muscle, or peripheral motor or sensory nervous system. Patients are well able to compensate for leg joint arthritis by limping, can learn to walk with prosthetic limbs, can waddle with severe proximal muscle weakness, and compensate for foot drop due to peripheral nerve lesions. Ataxia due to loss of proprioceptive, visual, or vestibular feedback usually leads to cautious walking. All these conditions produce a major threat to independent walking only when associated with other middle- or high-level disorders of gait which impair the normal compensatory mechanisms.

Middle-level gait disorders

In these, disease of the pyramidal tract, cerebellum, or basal ganglia interferes with the normal cerebral cortical mechanisms for maintaining equilibrium and implementing locomotor control. Cerebellar ataxia causes inaccurate striding and postural adjustment mechanisms. Early Parkinson's disease and pyramidal tract lesions impair postural responses. Once again, it is only when such disorders are very severe in themselves, or are conjoined with another gait disorder, that walking ability is completely abolished.

High-level gait disorders

These are the least well understood, and attract a variety of confusing descriptive labels. Most commonly they are known as gait apraxias. They reflect disease of those frontal lobe mechanisms responsible for selecting postural responses and locomotor behaviour suitable for the particular requirements of the patient at that moment. Manifestations of these disorders, and disabilities caused by them, vary widely between patients. Most usually they occur in the elderly, or in those with acquired bilateral disease of the frontal lobes due to ischaemia or demyelination. They involve varying combinations of the following features:

- cautious small steps (*marche à petits pas*) on a slightly wide base, and with careful walking round corners;

- poor postural responses with a tendency to fall backwards; inability to stand up, or to maintain balance whilst standing or sitting;

- inability to organize leg and trunk movements to keep the feet under the centre of gravity, and tangling of their feet on attempted cornering;

- gait ignition failure.

Walking sticks

These are helpful in the earlier stages of many walking disorders, before walking tripods, Zimmer frames, or even wheelchairs become required. Although walking sticks serve a valuable role for turning a patient's unstable bipedal gait into a more stable tripod, they do have three other main uses. First, when striding, they can take the weight off a painful joint. Second, walking sticks signal to the outside world that someone with an unsteady gait is not simply drunk. Third, many patients with frontal gait disorders, and Parkinsonism, find that walking is easier if they can concentrate on a rhythmically recurring feature such as paving stone cracks, or the tip of their walking stick repeatedly placed ahead.

Falls

A third of elderly patients fall each year. Many of them injure themselves significantly, particularly by fracturing their hips. Such injuries are an important cause of temporary or permanent disability, and sometimes death. Furthermore, such injuries may temporarily or permanently worsen the disability due to a pre-existing gait disorder.

Gait disorders are a leading cause of falls, particularly the high-level disorders that are particularly common in the elderly. Many such gait disorders are slowly progressive, and presumably reflect non-specific neurodegenerative disease. Stepwise progression of gait disorders may be due to cerebrovascular disease, sometimes known as atherosclerotic Parkinsonism, and should prompt consideration of measures to prevent further small strokes. The gait disorder of Parkinson's disease may improve with dopaminergic treatment, although the associated impairment of postural adjustment mechanisms often responds less well than the bradykinesia. Patients with gait disorders due to spinal cord disease should be investigated for potentially operable compressive cervical spondylitic radiculopathy. Rapidly evolving high-level gait disorders can reflect potentially operable structural cerebral disease, such as frontal meningiomas, subdural haematomas, obstructive hydrocephalus, or normal pressure hydrocephalus.

Of course there are many other causes of falls in the elderly, including fainting. Poor vision and poor illumination can lead to trips over environmental hazards. **Postural hypotension** is an important cause of falls in the elderly, often being precipitated by antihypertensive and vasodilator drugs. **Drop attacks** are momentary losses of postural tone whilst standing, without any loss of awareness of consciousness, and usually the patient is aware of falling before hitting the ground. The cause of drop attacks is not known; most patients will have only a handful of such attacks in their life before they resolve spontaneously.

Movement disorders

Abnormal movements

Chorea

Chorea is like an involuntary 'dancing' or fidgeting movement involving flexion and extension of the limb joints. Patients sometimes disguise these movements as mannerisms—for instance, bringing up the dancing hand to scratch the face. **Chorea** is an important feature of **Huntington's disease** (Chapter 30, p. 178) in which it is combined with dementia. It occasionally occurs in **pregnancy** (chorea gravadarum), and after streptococcal infections (Sydenham's chorea). Chorea is a common side-effect of dopaminergic drugs in patients with long-established Parkinson's disease.

Athetosis

Athetosis is a slow writhing movement around the long axis of the limb. It can be associated with chorea in Huntington's disease or as a side-effect of dopaminergic drugs in Parkinson's disease. Athetoid cerebral palsy results from perinatal brain injuries due to anoxia or the kernicterus associated with severe neonatal jaundice.

Dystonia

A dystonic limb is held stiffly in an odd posture because of co-contraction of agonist and antagonist muscles. Typically, **focal dystonia** produces stiff inturning of a foot and may follow injuries. **Dystonia musculoram deformans** is a rare inherited and generalized disabling dystonia. Temporary dystonic reactions may follow administration of dopamine antagonist drugs, such as phenthiazines or metoclopramide. These often take the form of alarming **occulogyric crises**, in which the head and eyes deviate uncontrollably in one direction, usually upwards.

Tremor

Tremor is a rapid vibratory movement which is usually noticed in the fingers and hand. Everyone has a **physiological tremor** at 6–8 Hz, which is usually invisible unless brought out by anxiety, thyrotoxicosis, antidepressant drugs, or with ageing. **Benign essential tremor** is an underdamped physiological tremor which can be dominantly inherited and typically suppressed by alcohol. It usually responds well to beta-blocker drugs. **Rest tremor** is typical of Parkinson's disease and usually takes the form of pill-rolling finger and thumb movements. **Intention tremor** occurs in cerebellar or sensory ataxia. Ataxia is not a tremor in the sense of being an uncontrollable rhythmic vibration. Rather it is a series of movements each correcting for the inaccuracy, or dysmetria, of the preceding movement. Head tremor is known as **titubation**, can be NO–NO or YES–YES in type, and can be an annoying feature of old age.

Myoclonus

Myoclonic jerks are sudden shock-like or startle movements of the whole limb. They occur in all of us when suddenly frightened, or when falling asleep. Pathological myoclonus occurs in juvenile myoclonic epilepsy, in anoxic brain damage, and in the progressive dementing illness Creutzfeldt–Jakob disease.

Parkinson's disease

Parkinson's disease is a progressive neurodegenerative disorder producing varying combinations of **bradykinesia**, **rest tremor**, **rigidity**, and **loss of postural adjustment**.

Causes

We do not know the cause of idiopathic Parkinson's disease, although an environmental toxin(s) is suspected. Most patients are older than 55 years. Some cases follow viral encephalitis, particularly in younger patients. However, **post-encephalitic Parkinsonism** has occurred only rarely since the influenza pandemic of 1918. Dopamine antagonist drugs, such as haloperidol or phenothiazines cause drug-induced **Parkinsonism** with bradykinesia and rigidity.

Pathology

Idiopathic Parkinson's disease results from degeneration of the dopamine-secreting **substantia nigra** neurons which project from the mid-brain to the corpus striatum. The substantia nigra loses its pigment in Parkinson's disease (Fig. 26.1) and the affected neuronal cell bodies show a characteristic eosinophilic cytoplasmic inclusion known as the **Lewy body**.

Clinical features

Initially Parkinson's disease is mild and patients merely notice a slight rest tremor of one hand or awkward or slow manipulations when doing buttons or playing the piano. If the dominant hand is affected, the writing becomes smaller and peters out within words—**progressive micrographia** (Fig. 26.2).

Other **bradykinetic** (i.e. slow movement) features that appear later include loss of facial expression, slowness in starting walking, delay in initiating swallowing, a monotonous weak voice, and loss of arm-swing whilst walking. The posture and gait are very characteristic (Fig. 26.3) with a hunched body, difficulty in getting going, loss of arm swing, slightly flexed arms, and a

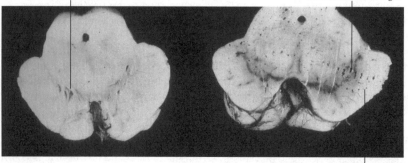

Loss of substantia nigra pigmentation in Parkinson's disease

Normal substantia nigra

Fig. 26.1 Depigmented substantia nigra in Parkinson's disease (left) compared with a normal midbrain (right).

Cerebral peduncle

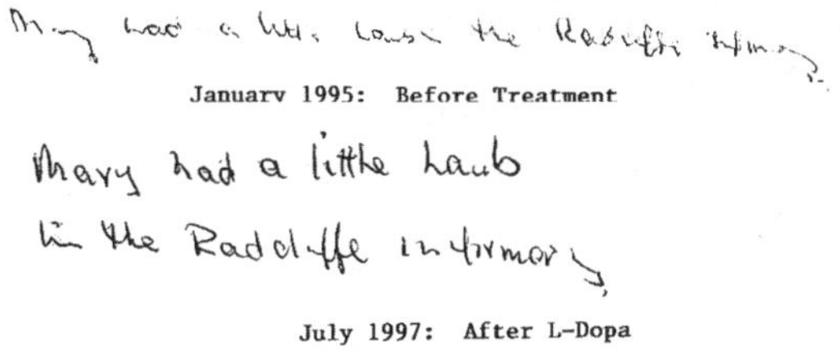

Tremor occurs at rest and usually consists of involuntary pill-rolling movements of the thumbs and forefingers. The muscular rigidity is unyielding or 'lead-pipe'. Rigidity with a superimposed tremor is called **cog-wheel rigidity**. This is best sought by holding the patients fingertips and feeling for resistance and tremor as you flex and extend the wrist and fingers (see Fig. 2.24, p. 19).

Loss of postural adjustment mechanisms cause patients to fall because they cannot recover from stumbles. To avoid falls, patients with Parkinson's disease should be advised to reorganize their homes so as to minimize the risk of tripping over furniture or carpet edges. Falling and fracturing an osteoporotic hip can be the beginning of the end for a patient with established Parkinson's disease.

Many patients with Parkinson's disease are troubled by **depression**, and some develop a mild **dementia**. Ultimately, patients with Parkinson's disease can become chair-bound, racked by tremor, may suffer malnutrition from dysphagia, and may die of aspiration pneumonia. But in many patients it is a slowly progressive disorder of old age, which does not cause overwhelming disability during the natural span of life.

Treatment

Replacement therapy for the dopamine deficiency of Parkinson's disease was one of the first successful treatments for a disabling neurological disorder. L-**dopa** is given orally, and later converted to dopamine within the brain by dopa decarboxylase. The L-dopa is normally combined with a peripheral **dopa decarboxylase inhibitor** (benserazide or carbidopa). This inhibitor does not cross the blood–brain barrier and prevents L-dopa from being converted to dopamine in the circulation before it enters the brain. If given without a decarboxylase inhibitor L-dopa causes the severe systemic dopaminergic side-effects of nausea and postural hypotension.

L-dopa improves symptoms in most patients with Parkinson's disease, sometimes dramatically. It particularly helps the bradykinesia. L-dopa is not a cure, but merely improves symptoms for some years. Larger doses of L-dopa are required as the underlying disease progresses, and this often induces involuntary movements, such as chorea, athetosis, or dystonia. These dyskinetic side-effects may be helped by amantidine, subcutaneous apomorphine infusions, or functional neurosurgery. Patients with advanced Parkinson's disease often start responding unpredictably to L-dopa, so-called 'on–off' phenomena. L-dopa may eventually

January 1995: Before Treatment

July 1997: After L–Dopa

Fig. 26.2 Micrographia in Parkinson's disease.

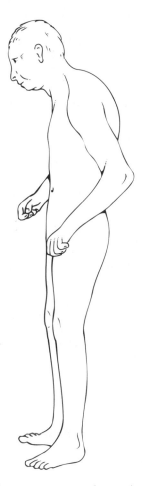

Fig. 26.3 A Parkinsonian stance. Note the typical posture, with flexed elbows and pill-rolling fingers.

pill-rolling tremor of finger and thumb. After a shuffling start the stride length gets longer and longer as though the patient is about to break into a run. Typically Parkinsonian patients 'get stuck' as they try to walk through an open doorway even though there is no physical obstruction.

become less effective in patients with severe and long-standing Parkinson's disease. If so, **direct-acting dopamine agonists** such as bromocriptine may help; indeed, increasingly these are being used earlier in the disease. Parkinsonian tremor responds less well to L-dopa than bradykinesia. Severe tremor may respond to centrally acting **anticholinergics** such as benzhexol, or even to stereotactic thalamotomy.

Falls, poor bulbar function, and dementia are particular problems in many with advanced Parkinson's disease. Unfortunately, the current treatments are relatively ineffective for these.

CASE 26.1 'A WINK'S AS GOOD AS A NOD'

A young housewife had been aware of 'live wires' around her right eye for some years. Sometimes these would cause the eyelid to blink involuntarily. They did not concern her until she went to her bedroom to review the installation of a fitted wardrobe. After looking at her intensely for a moment or two, the young carpenter approached embarrassingly closely, winking at her enthusiastically as he did so. Realizing that her symptom was giving confusing emotional signals, she sought medical advice. Neurological examination merely showed mild right hemifacial spasm sometimes leading to partial eye closure, and occasionally twitching of the corner of the mouth. Her mild hemifacial spasm was treated effectively by botulinum toxin injection of the periocular facial muscles.

Comment

- Hemifacial spasm is not a medically sinister condition, being either idiopathic, or due to irritation of the facial nerve intracranially by an aberrant loop of artery.

- Although anticonvulsant drugs can be effective in controlling hemifacial spasm, the most effective treatment is with repeated injections of low-dose botulinum toxin into the symptomatic muscles. This provided excellent symptom relief in this patient.

- Botulinum toxin, or botox, is derived from *Clostridium botulinum*. It acts presynaptically to prevent the release of acetylcholine at the neuromuscular junction and other cholinergic synapses. Botox has a wide variety of therapeutic uses for spasticity and movement disorders, for cosmetic reduction of facial wrinkles, and for preventing excessive sweating. Its effects last approximately 2 months before repeat administration is required; dosages are calculated so as to avoid weakening muscles outside the immediate vicinity of the injection site.

CASE 26.2 'SNORTS AND HEAD JERKS'

For 6 years a 24-year-old storeman had involuntarily jerked his head and made guttural noises. His head thrusts were more frequent under stress. More recently he had begun sniffing loudly and emphatically, and would make animal-like snorts and grunts and throat clearings, particularly at the beginning of sentences. His personality was somewhat obsessional in attention to detail and routine. Profound social disability had resulted, and apart from the necessity of going to work, he had avoided leaving his house for about 6 months.

Neurological examination was normal apart from the above-mentioned tics. To diminish these embarrassing tics due to his Gilles de la Tourette syndrome, he tried a centrally acting dopamine antagonist. Although this did not eliminate the tics, it reduced their occurrence to a much more tolerable level, allowing him to lead a fuller social life. However, their reduction left him feeling inwardly nervous and tense, a bottled-up feeling that he would sometimes relieve by stopping the drug for the weekend.

Comment

* Tics are common, particularly in boys before and during adolescence. They consist of repetitive movements or vocalizations. Generally they disappear spontaneously within a few months or years, and do not produce much embarrassment, except perhaps to the child's parents.

* Gilles de la Tourette syndrome is not uncommon. Its milder forms may go largely unnoticed, consisting of stereotyped throat clearings or gestures.

* The more severe forms involve repetitive gestures or vocalizations, which are often obscene or refer to excretions, so called coprolalia. Ritualistic behaviour patterns may occur. Some patients sport unusually exhibitionistic tattoos. Many are obsessional.

* To varying extents, most tics are voluntarily controllable. However, in Gilles de la Tourette syndrome this requires a very considerable effort of will and concentration. Voluntary or pharmacological inhibition of tics may make patients feel anxious and 'bottled-up' despite the obvious social benefits.

* All of us have a distinctive range of mannerisms of speech, gesture, facial expression, and gait. These are an important aspect of how we express our different personalities. It can be difficult to distinguish abnormal tics from normal and habitual mannerisms of the more eccentric variety.

* Tics and mannerisms attract the status of a disease if they are repetitive, stereotyped, or bizarre. Furthermore, they will be unrelated to, or intrude upon the ongoing conversation or social interaction. Most of us exhibit odd mannerisms or characteristics under profound stress or excitement, and Gilles de la Tourette syndrome may be an extreme of a normal continuum. A fascinating area of human psychology.

CHAPTER 27

Stroke

Chapter contents

Types of stroke

A stroke is a sudden neurological disturbance due to blockage or bursting of a brain blood vessel. There are three main types.

1 **Ischaemic stroke** due to blockage of a brain artery by an embolus or by thrombosis. If the neurological deficit lasts for more than 24 hours it is a **completed stroke**. If it lasts for less than 24 hours it is a **transient ischaemic attack (TIA)**.

2 **Haemorrhagic stroke** due to intracerebral haematoma.

3 **Subarachnoid haemorrhage** due to rupture of a blood vessel into the cerebrospinal fluid within the subarachnoid space.

Ischaemic stroke

Mortality due to ischaemic stroke is steadily declining in western countries. Yet it remains a huge cause of irreversible long-term disability, which affects many of working age. Most ischaemic stroke is due to **emboli** blocking a cerebral artery (Fig. 27.1). A smaller proportion is due to thrombosis, usually in those taking oral contraceptives, with a blood coagulation abnormality, or with pre-existing disease of small brain arteries. CT or MRI brain scan will usually show the infarct, although the appearance may not be evident within the 24 hours after onset. The main purpose of investigation is to detect potentially treatable causes so as to minimize the risk of further TIAs or completed strokes. But in many patients with stroke all the investigations are normal.

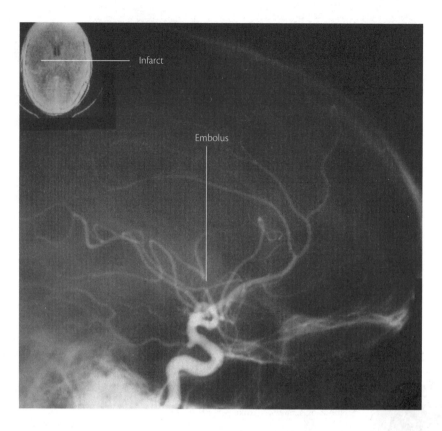

Fig. 27.1 A small embolus from the heart blocking a branch of the middle cerebral artery on an angiogram. The area of cerebral infarction is shown on the inset CT scan.

Emboli usually come from an internal carotid artery stenosed by atheroma. Sometimes emboli come from a heart affected by mitral valve disease, right to left shunts, bacterial endocarditis, mural thrombosis following myocardial infarction, or more commonly by isolated atrial fibrillation. The most important aspects of examining patients with ischaemic stroke consist of auscultation of the carotid artery for a bruit, indicative of stenosis, listening to the heart for valvular lesions, and taking the pulse to detect arrhythmia.

Carotid stenosis can be imaged non-invasively by ultrasound (carotid duplex) scans, by magnetic resonance angiography or by spiral CT. These techniques are replacing dye-injection angiography (Fig. 27.2), which carried a 1–2 per cent risk of causing or worsening an ischaemic deficit. **Echocardiography** will detect structural heart lesions.

Generally, ischaemic stroke is commonest in those who are diabetic, hypertensive, smoke, or have polycythemia.

Ischaemic stroke syndromes

Ischaemic stroke or TIA comes on suddenly and causes loss of function in the affected territory of the brain (Fig. 27.3).

The common stroke syndromes are:

1 A **middle cerebral artery stroke** causes contralateral **hemiparesis**, which will be noted immediately. If the left hemisphere is affected, **aphasia** may not be noted until the patient next speaks, reads, or listens.

2 A **posterior cerebral artery stroke** causes contralateral **homonymous hemianopia**, which may not be noted until the patient next tries to read, walk through doorways, or drive a car.

3 A **basilar artery stroke** affecting the brainstem causes varying combinations of **diplopia, ataxia, facial weakness**, and **altered facial sensation**. Emboli blocking the origin of both posterior cerebral arteries at the **top of the basilar** produce complete blindness (Fig. 27.5). Basilar artery occlusion can lead to unconsciousness, which is generally an unusual symptom of ischaemic stroke.

4 A stroke in the territory of the **posterior inferior cerebellar artery**, which is a branch of the vertebral artery, causes cerebellar infarction with **vertigo** and **ipsilateral cerebellar ataxia**.

5 **Lacunar infarcts** are small areas of damage deep within the cerebral hemispheres due to blockage of

Occasionally other vascular territories of the brain are affected by ischaemic stroke; for instance, an anterior cerebral artery infarction produces weakness of the contralateral leg.

A large infarct may swell over the next few days causing increasing neurological deficit, and eventually coma and death. Large middle-cerebral artery or basilar artery infarcts are especially likely to be fatal.

Treatment of ischaemic stroke

There are three aspects to treating stroke or TIA: acute measures, rehabilitation, and treatment of risk factors so as to prevent a further stroke.

Acute measures

The challenge of acute treatment of ischaemic stroke is to unblock the artery and restore perfusion before brain tissue has died. In reality, this window of opportunity is no more than a few hours at best, and falls well short of the time it usually takes to admit stroke patients to hospital. Immediate aspirin or heparin therapy slightly decreases the risk of early stroke recurrence, and of potentially fatal pulmonary embolism, but at the cost of haemorrhagic transformation of the stroke, particularly in the case of heparin. Intravenous thrombolitic therapy may have a modest overall benefit if given within 3 hours of stroke onset, but also carries the risk of haemorrhagic transformation of the infarct.

Early admission to specialist stroke units improves survival and outcome. Of particular importance are attention to treating pneumonia and other infections, preventing venous thrombosis with compression stockings to prevent pulmonary embolism, feeding and hydration, and regular turning to avoid pressure sores.

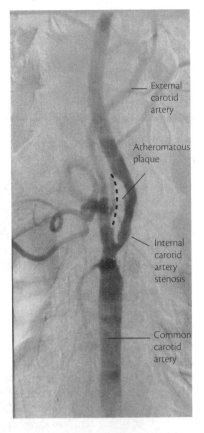

Fig. 27.2 A carotid angiogram showing stenosis of the proximal internal carotid artery.

the small penetrating arteries. They may constitute a quarter of all ischaemic strokes, although often silent and undetected. Hemiplegia may occur if they affect the internal capsule. Dementia can result from multiple lacunar infarcts.

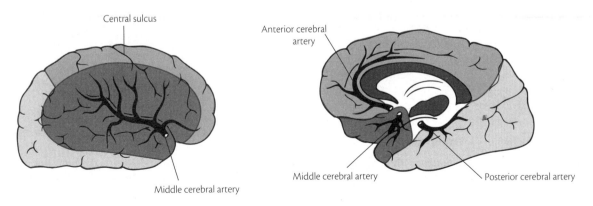

Fig. 27.3 The areas of the cerebral hemispheres supplied by the anterior, middle, and posterior cerebral arteries.

Rehabilitation

Rehabilitation can only maximize what function remains beyond the permanent deficit of a completed stroke. **Hemiplegic** patients usually learn to walk rather awkwardly once their paralysed leg has developed sufficient spasticity to bear weight. Incomplete **aphasics** recover some language abilities particularly if intelligent and helped by a talkative and well-motivated family, and guided by a speech therapist. Patients with a permanent **hemianopia** are not permitted to drive, and may find it difficult to read again. **Neglect** due to right parietal infarction can be phenomenally disabling.

Preventative treatments

Primary prevention aims to reduce stroke in the 'at-risk' population. Secondary prevention is particularly important in those who have had a warning TIA or small completed stroke but have not been permanently disabled by a large completed stroke.

Any general **risk factors** such as hypertension, diabetes mellitus, smoking, or polycythemia should be treated. Particular benefit comes from treating hyperlipidaemia with statin drugs.

Aspirin 150 mg daily should be given for life. This cuts the risk of future stroke or TIA by 20 per cent. The mechanism of the benefit is unknown, but may result from altering the prostaglandin metabolism involved in thrombosis. Patients unable to tolerate aspirin can use clopidogrel.

Surgical endarterectomy for a symptomatic carotid artery more than 70 per cent stenosed. But endarterectomy is a risky investment against further stroke. The operation itself carries a 5–10 per cent risk of death or stroke, but cuts down the risk of stroke thereafter. Thus, the overall risk only improves after the second or third postoperative year.

Cardiac emboli: cardiac surgery may be required for shunts and some valvar lesions. Warfarin anticoagulation reduces the risk of further stroke in isolated atrial fibrillation, in atrial fibrillation complicating mitral stenosis, and for mural thrombus complicating myocardial infarction. Anticoagulation has no proven role in primary stroke prevention except when there is a cardiac source of emboli.

Assessing treatments

There are two ways of considering the benefit of treatments used in neurological practice.

1 **Symptom reversal**. Many treatments show benefit by reversing or preventing an obvious symptom. Examples include drugs to prevent migraine or epileptic attacks, L-dopa to improve Parkinson's disease, or immunomodulatory drugs to reverse disability in neuromuscular disease. In such cases, usually both patient and physician can make a reasonably confident assessment of whether the treatment has helped that particular patient's symptoms. The drug can be stopped if there is inadequate response.

2 **Statistical benefit**. Increasingly, neurology uses therapies that are known to have a statistical benefit for a population of patients with a particular disease. But you never know whether the treatment has benefited the individual patient in front of you. Often it is unclear whether such treatments confer some degree of benefit on all patients, or whether they selectively benefit only a subpopulation. Examples include the use of beta interferon to reduce the relapse rate in multiple sclerosis, the use of riluzole in motor neuron disease, and the various approaches to primary and secondary prevention of stroke.

Crude statistical descriptions of changes in incidence and prevalence have little practical meaning for patients. So how best to assess the value of a preventative treatment, and describe its level of benefit in meaningful terms to the patient and other doctors? Refined statistical descriptions such as the **odds ratio** (± 95% confidence intervals; or ± 2 standard deviations) have been crucially valuable in showing whether risk factors or interventions are significant at the 5 per cent level. The odds ratio has particular value for comparing the impact of different variables or treatments. It also allows statistical overview of a pool of different randomized trials to provide **meta-analysis**.

Although the odds ratio expresses the **relative risk reduction** to be gained from a treatment, it does not provide a straightforward notion of **absolute risk reduction**. Indeed, treatment trials showing very similar relative risk reductions may have widely differing levels of absolute risk reduction. For patients, who generally have an unsophisticated grasp of statistics, it is the absolute risk reduction that is of interest. For this reason, the notion of '**number needed to treat** (to prevent one event)' is becoming popular, as are the notions of 'numbers needed to harm one (side-effect)' or 'number needed to screen (to detect one tumour)'. The number needed to treat corresponds to 100/absolute risk reduction.

If one applies this methodology to the prevention of one stroke after 5 years of treatment:

- 25 elderly patients need to be treated for **hypertension**;

- ◆ 40 TIA or stroke patients need to receive **aspirin**;

- ◆ 67 patients with established vascular disease, or asymptomatic patients with at least one risk factor for vascular disease (e.g. diabetes, hypertension) need to be treated with cholesterol-lowering **statin** drugs;

- ◆ 8 patients with recently symptomatic severe carotid stenosis need to undergo **carotid endarterectomy**.

These notions enable patients, doctors, and health economists to make more meaningful overall decisions about the likely benefit of a treatment, taking into account severity of side-effects and costs. The main practical challenge for doctors is to have the relevant statistic at one's fingertips, or in mind, whilst advising the patient.

Haemorrhagic stroke

The neurological deficit comes on less abruptly with haemorrhagic stroke than with ischaemic stroke. Headache is more likely. Haemorrhagic stroke is much less common than ischaemic stroke, and is immediately visible on CT scan (see Fig. 7.6, p. 54). The haemorrhage usually occurs deep within the cerebral hemisphere in hypertensives or those with coagulation disorders. Recurrent superficial haematomas in different parts of the cerebral cortex occur in a form of amyloid degeneration of cortical blood vessels in the elderly. There is little that can be done to influence the outcome of haemorrhagic stroke apart from promptly reversing any coagulation deficit. Surgical evacuation of the haematoma does not help in haemorrhages affecting the cerebral hemispheres, but can be life-saving if a cerebellar haemorrhage causes acute obstructive hydrocephalus or threatens to compress vital cardiorespiratory centres in the brainstem.

Subarachnoid haemorrhage

Subarachnoid haemorrhage is due to a brain blood vessel suddenly bursting and bleeding into the cerebrospinal fluid of the subarachnoid space. The headache is severe and comes on instantaneously 'like being hit on the head'. Subarachnoid haemorrhage may be provoked by exertion, sexual intercourse, or while straining. Immediate death occurs in about one-third. Another third become unconscious and have a high risk of dying or developing a permanent neurological deficit. The remaining third usually do well as long as re-bleeding is prevented. During the hours immediately following rupture, those with mild subarachnoid haemorrhage are conscious but may be slightly drowsy. Those with more severe subarachnoid haemorrhage will have focal deficits such as hemiplegia, be stuporose, comatose, or may become brain dead. Meningeal irritation by subarachnoid blood produces photophobia (dislike of bright lights) and neck stiffness (see Fig. 28.1, p. 168).

Diagnosis

Subarachnoid haemorrhage usually shows clearly on CT scan, with blood in the cortical sulci, cerebral ventricles, and around the base of the brain and brainstem (Fig. 27.4). Lumbar puncture proves the diagnosis if the CT scan is not diagnostic. The cerebrospimal fluid contains thousands of red blood cells per mm³, and the supernatant will be xanthochromic (straw-coloured) after centrifugation. **Xanthochromia** is due to altered haemoglobin pigments released from lysed red cells.

Causes

There are three main causes of subarachnoid haemorrhage:

1 **Rupture of an aneurism** on the **circle of Willis** or basilar artery (Fig. 27.5) accounts for about 80 per cent of the cases.

The aneurism is localized by angiography (Fig. 27.6). It is usually impossible to predict the location of the aneurism on simple clinical grounds. Sometimes posterior communicating artery aneurisms press on the adjacent third nerve, causing an oculomotor nerve palsy. Aneurisms can be treated by craniotomy and **surgical clipping**, or by **interventional angiography**, which places a wire coil within the aneurismal sac to promote thrombosis and obliteration (see Fig. 20.5, p. 125).

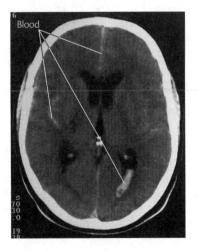

Fig. 27.4 Subarachnoid haemorrhage showing blood in the left sylvian fissure, the occipital horn of the right lateral ventricle, and in the interhemispheric fissure (CT scan, unenhanced).

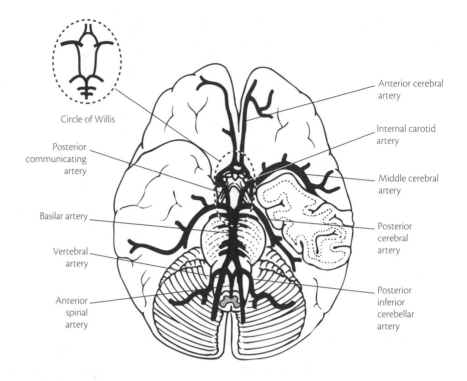

Fig. 27.5 The circle of Willis and the other arteries at the base of the brain.

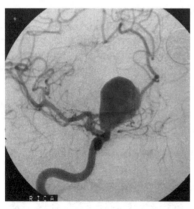

Fig. 27.6 A giant aneurism of the terminal carotid artery (arteriogram). This same aneurism is also shown in a CT scan (Fig. 7.1, p. 52).

2 **Rupture of an arteriovenous malformation** (AVM) accounts for about 5 per cent of cases (Fig. 27.7). AVMs have been present as a congenital anomaly since birth and may remain silent and undetected throughout life. Sometimes an AVM is detected because of epilepsy or focal neurological deficits. The risk of an AVM rupturing if untreated is roughly 2 per cent per annum. Obliteration by surgery, interventional angiography, and focused radiotherapy can be successful but such

treatments are sometimes avoided because of the high risk of creating a neurological deficit.

3 **No underlying vascular abnormality** is detected at angiography in about 15 per cent of cases. Many of these are youngish women who smoke and take the oral contraceptive tablet. Their subarachnoid haemorrhage is often mild and their prognosis is generally good.

Treatment

Treatment of subarachnoid haemorrhage involves two steps:

1 **Obliteration of the bleeding point** by surgery or by interventional radiology to prevent re-bleeding. In conscious patients without a serious focal deficit the aneurism can be obliterated within the first few days. Prior to surgery, strict bedrest minimizes the chance of a re-bleed.

2 **Preventing vasospasm**. Much of the delayed morbidity and mortality occurring in the days and weeks following subarachnoid haemorrhage is due to brain infarction resulting from vasospasm. The spasm is caused by vasoactive breakdown products derived from the decomposing subarachnoid blood. The risk of death is reduced by nimodipine, a calcium channel antagonist that penetrates the blood–brain barrier, and is thought to reduce vasospasm.

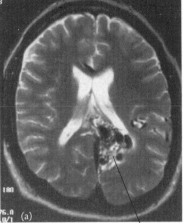
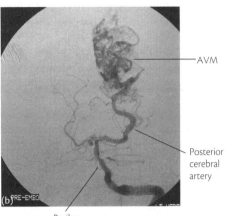

Fig. 27.7 (a) MRI showing an occipital lobe arteriovenous malformation (AVM) supplied by (b) a hypertrophied posterior cerebral artery (angiogram).

Occipital lobe AVM

AVM

Posterior cerebral artery

Basilar artery

CASE 27.1 'TREATABLE VISUAL LOSS'

A man in his 50s was referred by an ophthalmologist because of progressive loss of vision over 1 week. Initially things had looked intermittently washed out and later he had become unable to read easily, or to find his way around 'although I could have told someone else how to get there'. He also had episodes of numbness of an arm lasting a few minutes at a time, and intermittent difficulty finding words. A CT brain scan showed bilateral infarctions of the occipital lobes, thereby explaining his cortical visual loss. For 6 weeks he had had distressing and worsening head and neck pain. This raised the question of cerebral vasculitis, which was proved by the finding of increased lymphocyte count in his spinal fluid, and segmental narrowings of cerebral arteries on angiography (Fig. 27.8). General examination and microscopy of the urinary sediment revealed no evidence that this was part of a systemic vasculitis such as polyarteritis nodosa or Wegener's granulomatosis. Because of the severe and progressive nature of his cerebral symptoms, he was treated with cyclophosphamide which immediately stabilized his condition. This drug was tailed off over 6 months. He made a good recovery with only minor residual visual difficulties, and remained in remission thereafter.

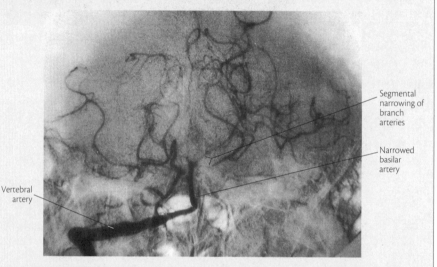

Fig. 27.8 Cerebral vasculitis. Vertebral arteriogram showing narrowings and obliterations of the basilar and posterior cerebral arteries and their branches.

Segmental narrowing of branch arteries

Narrowed basilar artery

Vertebral artery

Comment

- Occasionally cerebral infarction is due to disorders other than atherosclerosis, thrombosis, cholesterol emboli, or platelet emboli. Important examples include subacute bacterial endocarditis and vasculitis.

- Vasculitis is an inflammatory condition of the vessel wall which narrows and blocks arteries. It can be restricted to the cerebral arteries, producing a purely neurological syndrome as in this patient, or it can be part of a systemic arteritis which may involve the kidneys, skin, gastrointestinal tract, or respiratory tract. It can also be restricted to the cranial arteries outside the brain, called temporal (giant cell) arteritis (Chapter 20, p. 121), which can cause unilateral blindness.

- Diagnosing cerebral vasculitis is difficult. In this patient it was relatively easy because of the typical clinical, spinal fluid, and angiographic picture. Rapidly progressive symptoms in the territories of different cerebral arteries, the headache, and the inflammatory spinal fluid prompted cerebral angiography, which proved diagnostic. However, in some patients neurosurgical biopsy of the meninges may be necessary to prove the diagnosis.

- It is crucially important to diagnose and treat cerebral vasculitis promptly so as to prevent further irreversible cerebral damage. The definitive therapy is cyclophosphamide. But this must not be used lightly since it can produce dangerous bone marrow suppression, susceptibility to infections, haemorrhagic cystitis, and over the longer term, bladder cancer.

CASE 27.2 'WILL IT HAPPEN TO HIM AGAIN DOCTOR?'

A man in his 40s developed sudden severe pain in the left side of his neck and head, and so abandoned his evening gymnastics and went to sleep. Within hours he had become nauseated, and his wife found him to have a mixed dysphasia with a droopy left eyelid. Subsequent examination showed facial weakness and an extensor plantar response on the right. CT scan revealed left parietal infarction. Angiography showed a left internal carotid artery dissection (Fig. 27.9). He was started on antiplatelet therapy. It was decided to start anticoagulants only if he developed evidence of embolization from the distal stump of the dissected internal carotid artery. Fortunately this never occurred and his speech recovered reasonably well.

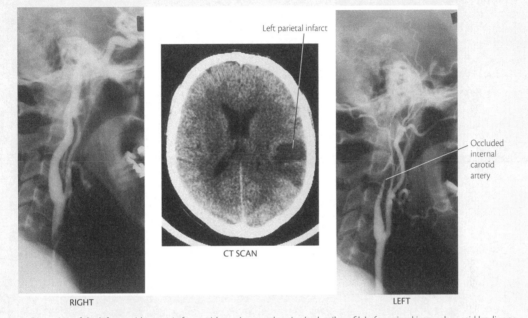

Left parietal infarct

CT SCAN

Occluded internal carotid artery

RIGHT

LEFT

Fig. 27.9 Dissection of the left carotid artery. Left carotid arteriogram showing 'rat's tail profile' of proximal internal carotid leading to complete occlusion; this should be compared with the normal right carotid artery. The resultant left parietal infarct, extending to the cortical surface, is shown in the CT scan.

Comment

◆ Arterial dissection is a relatively rare cause of ischaemic stroke. It can be caused by neck trauma or occur in those with inherited abnormalities of connective tissue. Blood tracks along a split in the arterial wall creating a false lumen. The artery becomes occluded by the haematoma within its wall and thrombosis and embolism may occur distally. Sometimes recanalization occurs by recommunication of the aneurism with the true arterial lumen.

◆ A patent circle of Willis may provide entirely adequate alternative cerebral perfusion, thereby avoiding cerebral infarction. Unfortunately this was not the case in this patient.

◆ Apart from the onset of neck pain during exertion, the other clue to the underlying cause of this patient's stroke was the presence of a left Horner syndrome. This reflected damage to the sympathetic plexus surrounding the dissected carotid artery.

◆ Will it happen again? Statistically, further dissections do eventually occur in a number of cases, for instance, in the other carotid artery. One must temper the need to provide a frank answer with the possibility of making patient and spouse fearful of returning to a rewarding life.

Neurological infection

Meningitis

Meningitis is an infection by bacteria, fungi, or viruses of the subarachnoid space, which is full of cerebrospinal fluid (CSF). It ranges from acute bacterial meningitis which may cause death within a few hours if untreated, to the very slow deterioration over weeks seen with fungal infections.

Typical meningitic symptoms are **headache, photophobia, fever**, and **progressive drowsiness** culminating in stupor or **coma**. Examination shows **neck stiffness** due to meningeal irritation (Fig. 28.1). Neck stiffness is difficult to elicit in frantic infants and children in whom it is often easier to put one arm behind the knees and the other behind the neck and to see if the chin can be touched to the knees.

Signs of focal neurological damage are unusual early on in meningitis, but may develop later when ischaemic and infective damage affects the substance of the brain.

In a patient without focal signs, you should proceed straight to a diagnostic lumbar puncture, so that antimicrobial treatment may be started without delay.

Any early focal sign in a meningitic patient, such as a hemiparesis or ocular palsy, should raise the question of a brain abscess and requires a brain scan. In a patient with focal signs there is the potential danger that the lumbar puncture will cause a pressure cone if there is an abscess. In this situation, blood cultures should be drawn, before giving a broad spectrum cephalosporin intravenously and then performing a brain scan.

Types of meningitis

Acute bacterial meningitis

Meningococcal meningitis (*Neisseria meningitidis*) is often epidemic and can cause death rapidly; it causes a dramatic purpuric skin rash in about half of cases. **Pneumococcal** meningitis (*Streptococcus pneumoniae*)

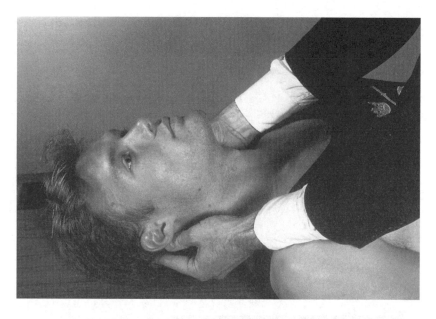

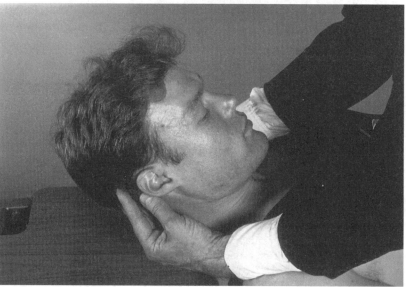

Fig. 28.1 Testing for neck stiffness in suspected meningitis or subarachnoid haemorrhage. You should remove the pillow, rest your wrists on the patient's shoulders, and use your fingers to flex the neck whilst assessing the degree of resistance.

often follows respiratory tract or sinus infections, or sometimes gains access via a post-traumatic spinal fluid leak through the ear or nose. *Haemophilus influenzae* meningitis often follows respiratory tract infections in children. **Neonatal** meningitis is usually due to *Escherichia coli* or Group B streptococci and often presents with a non-specific illness, convulsions, and a bulging fontanelle.

In acute bacterial meningitis the CSF shows thousands of polymorphonuclear white blood cells per mm^3, with a low CSF sugar concentration (i.e. less than half the blood sugar concentration). The Gram stain,

and later the bacterial culture, will guide specific antibiotic therapy. While awaiting bacterial diagnosis, a third-generation cephalosporin antibiotic should be given **intravenously** to cover the organisms commonly encountered in immunocompetent children and adults.

Subacute bacterial meningitis

This is usually **tuberculous** but can be due to *Listeria monocytogenes* in the immunosuppressed. Focal neurological abnormalities may occur in both. In tuberculosis these are due to tuberculomas in the brain,

TABLE 28.1 CSF in meningitis

Type of meningitis	Concentration in CSF		
	Polymorphs	Lymphocytes	Sugar
Acute bacterial (meningococcal, pneumococcal, *Haemophilus*)	++++	±	Low
Subacute bacterial (**TB**, *Listeria*)	++	++	Low
Chronic fungal	±	++	Low
Viral		+++	Normal
Malignant		+†	Low

† These "lymphocytes" are found to be malignant on cytology.

or tuberculous exudates involving the cranial nerves and brain blood vessels. *Listeria* often causes an associated brainstem encephalitis. In both types the CSF usually shows a mixture of lymphocytes and polymorphonuclear cells, with a low CSF sugar. Ziehl–Nielsen staining may immediately prove the infection is tuberculous.

Chronic fungal meningitis

Chronic fungal meningitis is usually due to *Cryptococcus neoformans*. This generally occurs in immunosuppressed patients such as transplant recipients or those with HIV infection. The CSF is lymphocytic, with a low sugar. Cryptococcal antigen may be detected in the CSF serologically; cultures may take weeks to become positive.

Viral meningitis

Viral meningitis presents as an acute illness but the patient is not as seriously ill as with bacterial meningitis. The CSF is lymphocytic with a normal sugar level. Recovery occurs spontaneously over a few days or weeks.

Malignant meningitis

Malignant meningitis may be confused with the more chronic forms of infective meningitis. It is usually due to adenocarcinoma from the breast or gastrointestinal tract, or to leukaemia or lymphoma. CSF cytology is diagnostic but sampling may need to be repeated two or three times to obtain a 'positive'. The CSF sugar is usually low in malignant meningitis.

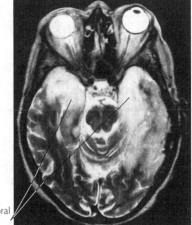

Medial temporal lobe oedema

Fig. 28.2 Herpes simplex encephalitis. Oedematous signal change in the medial temporal lobes; worse on the right (MRI).

Encephalitis

Encephalitis is a destructive inflammation of the brain substance usually caused by viruses. One form of encephalitis is **parainfectious** and caused by an indirect immunological consequence of a systemic viral infection; an example is the drowsiness or coma which can follow measles infection. The more serious forms of encephalitis are due to **direct viral infection** of the brain substance. These are often geographically restricted, for instance, the tick-borne forms of encephalitis in central Europe and Russia, or transmission of rabies by dog bites in endemic areas.

Herpes simplex encephalitis is the commonest form of severe encephalitis due to direct viral invasion. It is crucial to consider this diagnosis promptly since early administration of the specific antiviral drug **Acyclovir** greatly reduces death and long-term disability. Typically, a patient with herpes simplex encephalitis becomes confused, headachy, feverish and has seizures over a couple of days. The MRI brain scan (Fig. 28.2) may be normal, or show changes in the temporal lobe(s). The CSF shows up to a few hundred lymphocytes per mm^3. Acyclovir must be administered once the diagnosis is suspected. Brain biopsy to prove herpes infection is rarely justified given the effectiveness of acyclovir. Herpesvirus genome may be detected by a positive polymerase chain reaction (PCR) on CSF.

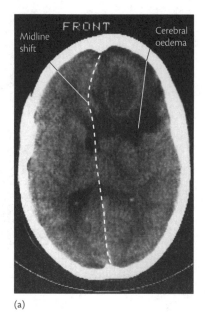

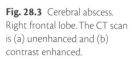

Fig. 28.3 Cerebral abscess. Right frontal lobe. The CT scan is (a) unenhanced and (b) contrast enhanced.

(a)

(b)

Brain abscess

Bacterial brain abscess results from either of the following:

1 infected emboli in patients who may have cyanotic congenital heart disease, or chronic lung sepsis such as bronchiectasis;

2 direct extension from an untreated infection of the middle ear or frontal sinuses.

Patients develop focal signs such as hemiparesis over a few days, associated with fever and drowsiness, and sometimes seizures. Death occurs due to a pressure cone if treatment is not initiated. Brain scans show a circular mass lesion with a contrast-enhancing capsule and considerable surrounding oedema (Fig. 28.3). Surgical drainage and antibiotic therapy arrest the infection. Permanent complications such as focal epilepsy or hemiparesis often remain.

Prion diseases

Creutzfeldt–Jakob disease of humans is caused by an infective proteinaceous particle called a **prion**, which contains no nucleic acid. The patient becomes progres-

sively **demented** with **ataxia** and **myoclonic jerkings** of the limbs and dies within 3–6 months. At autopsy the brain shows striking microscopic vacuolation due to lost neurons, known as **spongiform encephalopathy**. Although sometimes familial due to host prion gene mutations, Creutzfeldt–Jakob disease is usually sporadic. The mode of infection is not known, although transmission has occurred by neurosurgical instruments or pituitary hormones extracted from humans.

New variant Creutzfeldt–Jakob disease occurs in younger patients. Depression is often prominent from the outset, movement disorders overshadow dementia early on, there is less myoclonus, and a different neuropathological profile compared with normal Creutzfeldt–Jakob disease. This variant appeared as a result of the British population eating beef during the epidemic of bovine spongiform encephalopathy. **Bovine spongiform encephalopathy** followed the introduction of scrapie-infected material from sheep into the diet of cows, a normally herbivorous species.

Kuru is another form of spongiform encephalopathy occurring in the Fore highlanders of New Guinea and was transmitted by cannibalism.

Immunocompromised patients

There are many patients who have impaired immunity due to immunosuppressant drugs for preventing transplant rejection, chemotherapy for cancers, immunomodulation of autoimmune disorders, and HIV infection. All are vulnerable to neurological infection. But these are not the usual acute bacterial meningitis, herpes encephalitis, or pyogenic brain abscess. A wide range of organisms may occur, resistant strains are common, and choice of antibiotics is a specialist matter for infectious disease experts. The commoner infections are:

1 **Meningitis** is usually bacterial, due *Listeria*, tuberculosis, or fungal due to *Cryptococcus*.

2 **Focal cerebral abnormalities**, often multiple, are usually due to reactivation of the protozoan *Toxoplasma gondii*, the fungus *Aspergillus*, or the bacterium *Nocardia asteroides*. The differential diagnosis is from cerebral lymphoma, itself common in the immunocompromised, and usually an Epstein–Barr virus-driven B-cell tumour.

3 **Diffuse encephalopathy** is either viral, due to cytomegalovirus, or due to diffuse destruction of white matter, so-called progressive multifocal leucoencephalopathy, due to reactivation of papovavirus.

CASE 28.1 'NOT WHAT IT SEEMED, FORTUNATELY'

A patient with 'multiple cerebral metastases' was introduced with his CT scan at the end of a busy ward round. His smoker's cough and weight loss had provoked the clear implication that little diagnostic thought was necessary, given that time was short. In his 40s, he was a Caucasian odd-job man who had never travelled far from his birthplace in a British country town. His vision had blurred progressively for a month accompanied by headache worse in the morning. He had florid papilloedema and visual acuity reduced to 6/36 bilaterally. The right plantar response was equivocal. His memory seemed poor and he didn't talk spontaneously. CT scan showed multiple enhancing lesions throughout the brain surrounded by considerable oedema and some hydrocephalus (Fig. 28.4). Chest X-ray showed the extensive apical calcification and fibrosis of old tuberculosis but sputum cytology was negative for acid-fast bacilli. Because of lack of proof of underlying cancer, a right frontal lobe biopsy was arranged. This yielded two caseating granulomas, with giant cells and positive Ziehl–Nielson staining for acid-fast bacilli. Quadruple anti-tuberculous therapy produced a steady improvement over the next 6 months. Vision improved to 6/9 with resolution of the papilloedema, although some secondary optic atrophy developed. He returned to work successfully and remained well.

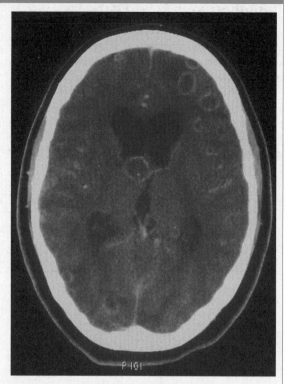

Fig. 28.4 Multiple cerebral tuberculomas, shown by contrast-enhanced brain CT scan. Note the deeply located tuberculoma causing hydrocephalus by interfering with drainage from the lateral ventricles.

Comment

- One needs to consider the possibility that any cerebral mass lesion could be infective, and therefore potentially curable. Bacterial cerebral abscess, tuberculoma, or toxoplasmosis can all produce brain scan appearances considered typical of brain tumour(s).

- Patients with multiple cerebral mass lesions, be they tumours or abscesses, may show a remarkable paucity of focal neurological signs. They may present with features of raised intracranial pressure, as did this patient, or with those of a generalized encephalopathy, such as confusion and tremulousness.

- Many brain infections are associated with particular geographical risk factors, or a known immunocompromised state. However, they can occur without either such predisposition, requiring a high degree of clinical suspicion for detection.

CASE 28.2 'RECURRING MENINGITIS'

A woman in her 40s was admitted with a few days of headache, neck stiffness, nausea, vomiting, and photophobia. Over the preceding 15 years she had had five identical such attacks. Always the CSF had been lymphocytic, with normal sugar content and negative examination for tuberculosis and fungi. By this sixth occasion, PCR testing for viral genomes had become available and showed that she had a meningeal infection with herpes simplex virus type II. The symptoms resolved completely within 2 days of starting the antiviral drug, acyclovir. It was concluded that her recurrent attacks of lymphocytic meningitis had been due to meningeal infection with reactivations of herpes simplex type II. Presumably this was not manifesting as the usual recurrent ulceration of the genitals, but of the caudal meninges, which receive the same sacral sensory root innervation. She was advised to take acyclovir tablets at the start of another typical attack, and did not need to be hospitalized for the condition again.

Comment

- Although lymphocytic meningitis occurs equally frequently to the more serious bacterial meningitis, only rarely is the causative virus identified.

- Lymphocytic meningitis due to viruses usually recovers well, and spontaneously. Yet it must be differentiated by CSF investigation from lymphocytic meningitis due to other serious conditions such as partially treated bacterial, tuberculous, or fungal forms of meningitis, and from malignant meningitis. A clue to all these other conditions is a low CSF sugar, but this is not invariable.

- Syndromes of recurrent lymphocytic meningitis have long been recognized, often called Mollaret's meningitis. This patient reminds us that many of these are now known to have a potentially treatable underlying herpesvirus infection. These periodically reactivate in much the same way as recurrent cold sores on the lips.

Head injury

Head injury is a common medical problem usually due to road traffic or industrial accidents. It may lead to brain death, permanent brain damage, post-traumatic epilepsy, or a prolonged post-traumatic syndrome. The incidence of head injury is decreasing because of improved statutory safety regulations such as safety belts and speed restrictions.

Grading severity

It is useful to grade the **severity** of head injury in terms of whether unconsciousness occurred, the length of the post-traumatic amnesia (loss of memory of subsequent events), whether focal brain damage occurred, and whether there is a skull fracture.

- **Mild**. Both unconsciousness and/or post-traumatic amnesia < 30 minutes.

- **Moderate**. Skull fracture and/or unconsciousness or post-traumatic amnesia > 30 minutes.

- **Severe**. > 24 hours unconsciousness or post-traumatic amnesia and/or focal brain damage or intracranial haematoma.

Intracerebral contusion or haematoma is particularly likely to affect the temporal or frontal lobes. These lobes get banged against protrusions on the inside of the skull if the head rotates during oblique impacts.

The principal worry after mild or moderate head injury is the delayed development of an extradural haematoma. These patients 'talk again then die'. Depressed skull fractures, and extradural or subdural haematomas may require prompt neurosurgical treatment. Patients with mild head injury are often managed as outpatients as long as someone responsible is available at home to supervise the next day or two.

Extradural haematoma

This feared complication is more likely if a skull fracture occurred, or if the head injury was severe. Typically the patient awakens from the concussion, and then becomes unconscious again as the extradural haematoma accumulates over the next 24 hours—after a '**lucid interval**'. The extradural haematoma accumulates between the dura mater and the skull due to laceration of the meningeal blood vessels (see Fig. 7.3, p. 54). As the haematoma accumulates, the patient rapidly becomes unconscious and will die from a pressure cone unless the haematoma is drained surgically. CT scan will identify on which side of the skull to carry out burr hole drainage. If faced with a rapidly expiring patient without a scan being available, the haematoma is most likely to be on the same side as the skull fracture. Furthermore, the pupil is often dilated on that side because of third nerve compression.

Subdural haematoma

Subdural haematoma collects between the dural and arachnoid layers of the meninges. It may be **acute** following head injury, in which case there will be a lucid interval and a fairly rapid decline resembling extradural haematoma. More often subdural haematoma has been chronically present for weeks or months. **Chronic** subdural haematoma may follow minor head injury in the elderly, in alcoholics, and those taking anticoagulants. Chronic subdurals often present rather non-specifically with variable headache, confusion, and drowsiness; the expected contralateral hemiparesis is often not detectable. CT scan shows fresh blood (white) in acute subdurals (Fig. 29.1). Isodense change in the clot of a chronic subdural haematoma may lead to it being indistinguishable from the brain and overlooked on CT scan. MRI scan is more sensitive in detecting subdural haematoma than CT scan. Chronic subdurals are often bilateral. Surgical drainage is required for larger haematomas, but often small ones can be managed conservatively and often resorb spontaneously.

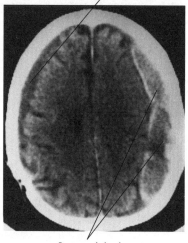

Old subdural collection

Recent subdural haematoma

Fig. 29.1 Bilateral subdural haematomas (CT scan). A small isodense subdural collection is present on the left and a larger fresher haematoma on the right.

Post-traumatic epilepsy

Over 10 per cent of those with severe head injury will develop epilepsy within 5 years. However, the risk after mild head injuries is barely greater than normal.

Post-traumatic syndrome

After mild or moderately severe head injuries, some patients are disabled by recurrent headaches, feelings of imbalance, depression, and mental dulling, which generally recover over 6 months to 3 years. There is no evidence that structural brain damage is responsible. Post-traumatic syndrome is commonly the subject of personal injury litigation. Sometimes malingering is alleged, but that is not the only explanation. Antidepressant drugs may speed recovery.

Neurogenetics

Genetic mechanisms

A huge variety of neurological diseases are genetic. Although each is rare, many cause serious disability, often long-term. The simple genetic principles of autosomal recessive, autosomal dominant, and sex-linked recessive inheritance underlie many of these neurological diseases. But we are aware also of diseases caused by variable length trinucleotide repeats and mutations of mitochondrial DNA.

Molecular genetic testing poses difficult **ethical problems** which must be thought through beforehand. For instance, if you are at risk of Huntington's disease, would you wish to undergo molecular genetic screening that would tell you for sure whether you will develop that severe, untreatable, and distressing disease?

And you might already have children and be aware that you have put them at risk. Or if you suffer from Charcot-Marie-Tooth disease, which often causes only mild leg weakness would you consider it necessary for your unborn fetus to be screened for the disease, with a view to selective abortion, given that Charcot-Marie-Tooth disease rarely causes overwhelming disability?

Autosomal recessive inheritance

Werdnig–Hoffman disease

Werdnig-Hoffman disease or infantile spinal muscular atrophy, is a typical example of classic Mendelian autosomal recessive inheritance. If both parents are heterozygous, on average one in four of their children will be affected. The incidence of Werdnig–Hoffman disease is 1:25,000 births. Most affected children die within their second year of progressive limb and bulbar weakness due to lower motor neuron degeneration. The responsible SMN gene on chromosome 5 has now been identified, with the prospect of offering prenatal diagnosis to affected families.

Autosomal dominant disorders

Gene reduplications: Charcot–Marie–Tooth disease

Charcot–Marie–Tooth is a dominantly inherited hypomyelinating disorder affecting peripheral nerves. It is present from early childhood, but is usually noted only in adulthood. Foot deformity with high arches (pes cavus) and muscle wasting and weakness below the knees, makes the legs look like 'inverted champagne bottles' (Fig. 30.1). The weakness progresses only slightly during life, rarely causes overwhelming disability, and affects the hands in only a third of patients. Charcot–Marie–Tooth disease is usually caused by re-duplication of a peripheral nerve myelin protein (PMP) gene on chromosome 17. This gene normally controls growth of the myelin spiral. Thus, double dosage of the gene inhibits myelin sheath growth, leading to a

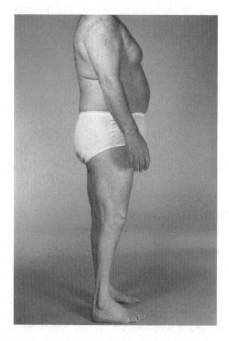

Fig. 30.1 Charcot–Marie–Tooth disease: inverted champagne bottle legs.

hypomyelinating neuropathy. Interestingly, when the PMP gene is deleted, uncontrolled overgrowth of myelin sheath occurs. This causes the condition of **hereditary liability to pressure palsies** of peripheral nerves, also dominantly inherited.

Expanded trinucleotide repeats: Huntington's disease

Huntington's disease is an autosomally dominantly inherited neurodegenerative disorder presenting in middle age with progressive dementia, psychiatric disturbance, and a choreiform movement disorder. The incidence is 1:10,000. The causative gene lies on chromosome 4 and encodes a protein called **Huntingtin** whose normal function remains unknown. The 5′ end of this gene contains a CAG trinucleotide repeat sequence containing 9–37 copies in normal people. Patients with Huntington's disease have 37 copies or more of this trinucleotide repeat. Measurement of the length of this repeat allows molecular genetic prediction of whether an individual will develop the disease, and of whether a fetus is carrying it. The greater the length of the repeat, the earlier the onset of the disease. The trinucleotide repeat is unstable, tending to get longer with successive generations. This explains why successive generations of a family may be affected at ever younger ages—a phenomenon known as anticipation. Similar expanded trinucleotide repeats are associated with the genes responsible for other neurodegenerative disorders presenting in middle age such as a form of motor neuron disease known as **X-linked bulbospinal neuronopathy**, an autosomal dominantly inherited muscle disease known as **myotonic dystrophy**, and a progressive cerebellar ataxia known as **Friedreich's ataxia**.

Sex-linked recessive disorders

Duchenne muscular dystrophy

Duchenne muscular dystrophy is an X-linked disorder which affects boys and weakens the leg, respiratory, and cardiac muscles. Most die by the age of 13 years. It is often suspected at an early age, when the boy is unable to stand up from the floor unless he uses his hands to 'walk' up the legs (**Gower's sign**). Calf muscle hypertrophy is typical both in Duchenne muscular dystrophy, and in the milder form affecting adults known as **Becker dystrophy** (Fig. 30.2).

Duchenne and Becker dystrophies are due to a range of mutations and deletions affecting the **dystrophin gene** on the X chromosome. Dystrophin is a protein

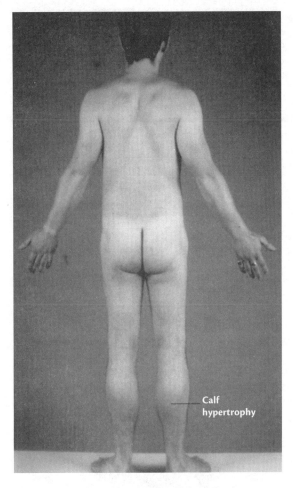

Fig. 30.2 Calf hypertrophy in Becker muscular dystrophy.

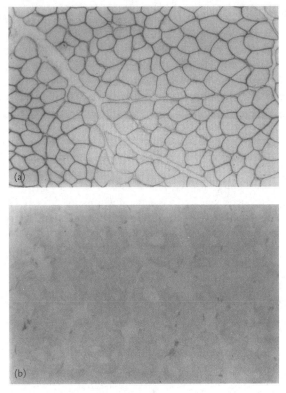

Fig. 30.3 Muscle biopsies stained for dystrophin. (a) Normal, showing uniform staining along the cell membranes. (b) Duchenne dystrophy, showing absence of dystrophin staining.

that normally anchors the actin filaments of the contractile apparatus into the muscle cell membrane. It is absent from the cell membrane in Duchenne dystrophy (Fig. 30.3). New mutations are frequent. Dystrophin gene analysis allows prenatal diagnosis in affected families.

Mitochondrial genome mutations

Mitochondrial DNA encodes many of the enzymes of the respiratory chain. Various mutations cause a diverse range of neurological disorders, which usually present in adulthood. These include:

1 **Leber's hereditary optic atrophy** in which one eye, followed by the other, goes blind permanently. Fundoscopy shows optic atrophy.

2 **Proximal muscle weakness**. Muscle biopsy shows copious mitochondria in 'ragged red' muscle fibres.

3 **MERRF**. *Myoclonic Epilepsy and Ragged Red* [muscle] *Fibres*.

4 **MELAS**. *Mitochondrial Encephalomyopathy, Lactic Acidosis and Stroke-like episodes*.

All these syndromes are transmitted through the maternal germline because we derive our mitochondria from the ovum. Mitochondria are sparse in spermatozoa.

CASE 30.1 'BEFORE MOLECULAR GENETIC TESTING'

A 60-year-old man was referred from another neuro-logist with an unusual question. 'Given that for more than 10 years he has had electromyographically con-firmed motor neuron disease affecting all four limbs, and the bulbar musculature, why was he still so well, and with so little disability?' Bulbar involvement usu-ally signifies a particularly poor prognosis with life expectancy measured in only a year or two. Examina-tion did reveal features of a motor neuron disease: a mild degree of wasting and weakness of the muscles of all four limbs, with some fasciculations, dysarthria, and a wasted and fasciculating tongue. But upper motor neuron signs, such as extensor plantars, were not present. These would have been expected were this the amyotrophic lateral sclerosis form of motor neuron disease. During history taking the patient showed the peculiar and distinctive physical sign of involuntary contractions of the lower facial muscles particularly after smiling or grimacing (Fig. 30.4). His wife had noted this feature across their breakfast table for some 20 years. The finding of gynaecomastia con-firmed that he had a form of slowly progressive bulbo-spinal motor neuron disease inherited as an X-linked recessive. At that time the molecular genetic test for this condition had not been invented. A cou-ple of years later, another man was referred with a similar syndrome, and the same unusual surname. He turned out to be the patient's estranged brother, thereby proving the genetic nature of the diagnosis. The patient and his brother were relieved to be re-assured that this carried a relatively benign prognosis compared with their gloomy expectations.

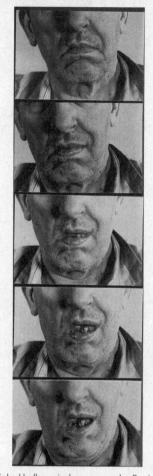

Fig. 30.4 X-linked bulbo-spinal neuronopathy. Persistence of lower facial muscular contractions in successive time frames after grimacing.

Comments

- There are a variety of different types of motor neuron degeneration, both sporadic and inherit-ed, with widely varying prognoses.

- X-linked bulbo-spinal neuropathy is an example of a neurological disorder due to an expanded trinucleotide repeat sequence within or adja-cent to a gene. In this case the repeat affects the androgen receptor gene.

- Gynaecomastia is characteristic. This can be de-tected by palpating the glandular tissue of the breast between thumb and fingers, rather than by rolling the breast against the chest wall with the flat of the hand, as you are taught for detect-ing tumours.

- X-linked recessive disorders are transmitted to males only through asymptomatic mothers. Thus, enquiry about affected ancestors is usually negative.

- If one of these brothers had a daughter it would raise the ethical difficulty of whether to screen any male fetuses for their carriage of this disorder should she elect to have children. But the disorder carries a near-normal life expectancy and the dis-ability is late and often not severe. This provokes thought about the value of prenatal screening.

Developmental disorders

Diseases of the infant's brain often come to light only when the parents sense that behaviour is failing to develop as anticipated. The variety of such disorders is enormous, and their precise diagnosis is the preserve of specialist paediatric neurologists. To detect developmental delay, you should ask the mother when the child mastered various skills (see Chapter 4). Often development has been uniformly slow throughout life, usually due to perinatal anoxic brain insults, cerebral palsy, or genetic disorders that affect the structure and wiring of the brain. Less often the rate of development slows down due to a new problem affecting the brain, such as the onset of hydrocephalus or a genetically determined lysosomal storage disorder that takes some years to produce clinical effects.

Cerebral palsy

Cerebral palsy is a term that covers a range of disorders, many still poorly understood. The central feature is **delayed motor development** that is non-progressive. Spastic diplegic (both legs), tetraplegic, hemiplegic, and athetoid forms occur. About a quarter of such patients never walk. Many also have mental retardation or epilepsy. Significant cerebral palsy occurs in about 1:500 live births.

The care of these children places a considerable burden on medical and social services, and on the anguished parents who know that their child will never develop normally. It is generally felt that birth anoxia is the leading cause of cerebral palsy. However, birth anoxia usually leads to babies either dying or surviving normally. Low-birth-weight babies of less than 1500 grams have a 25-fold increased rate of cerebral palsy. The recent increase in the incidence of spastic diplegic forms reflects the improved prospects of survival for low-birth-weight babies. It seems likely that much cerebral palsy will prove to be due to inherited and other congenital abnormalities of brain structure at a microscopic level.

Mental retardation

Mentally retarded children are backward in all aspects of development from birth, although motor functions can be less severely affected. As babies they are **late to smile**, and fail to develop the usual close bonds with their mother. Initially, questions of blindness or deafness may be raised as an explanation. Putting objects in the mouth and slobbering persist into adulthood. The attention span is poor. **Aggressive outbursts** may occur. Rhythmic **rocking** movements are common. Many are also **epileptic**. Language development is greatly delayed, and may never occur at all; many never develop beyond **screeches** and **grunts**. The head is often small and the body often underdeveloped for chronological age. The causes are incompletely understood but the following associations are common: small-for-dates babies, maternal rubella, cytomegalovirus, or toxoplasmosis infection during pregnancy, and a prior family history.

Autism

Even before the age of 2 years, children with autism are usually noted to lack social awareness and interaction. Often the behavioural repertoire is limited, particularly for imaginative play. Communication may be disturbed, particularly speech. Many such children have cognitive impairment, epilepsy, impaired motor control, or hyperactivity, meaning that the syndrome can overlap with mental retardation and cerebral palsy. The severity and clinical features vary immensely, making it more useful to think of '**the autistic spectrum of disorders**' rather than a single disease. A particularly noteworthy genetic form is known as **Asperger syndrome**, in which lack of social awareness and rigidity of behaviour are noteworthy, yet cognition is normal. Some people with this syndrome can be high achievers, often in a narrow area, and yet find it difficult to understand anyone else's perspective. It is at the mild end of the autistic spectrum that diagnosis becomes most difficult, being influenced by cultural perspectives, and parental expectations, and the wish for a label to explain and justify certain character traits.

Spina bifida

This occurs in 1:1000 births and can be familial. It is partially preventable by routine folic acid administration from the start of pregnancy. Screening for spina bifida during pregnancy involves high-resolution ultrasound imaging of the fetal spine and sampling the amniotic fluid for raised α-fetoprotein levels. Spina bifida is due to failure of the dorsal part of the primitive neural tube to fuse in the first few

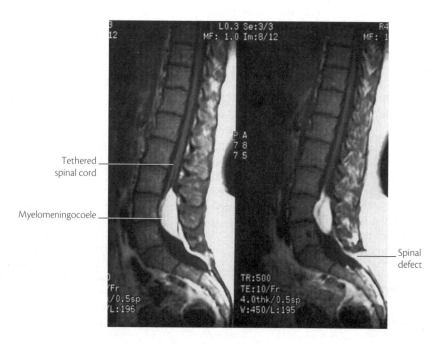

Tethered spinal cord

Myelomeningocoele

Spinal defect

Fig. 31.1 Spina bifida showing the myelomeningocele, tethered spinal cord, and the vertebral bone defect (MRI).

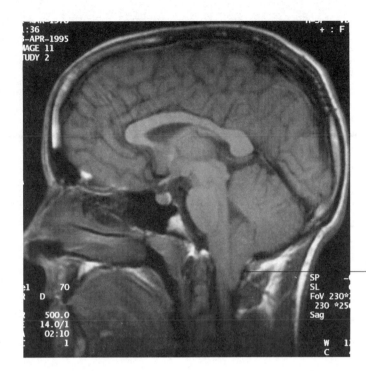

Fig. 31.2 A Chiari malformation of the cerebellar tonsils (MRI).

Tonsillar herniation through foramen magnum

weeks of embryonic and fetal life. Mild spina bifida is relatively common, usually causing no neurological problems. These mild forms known as **spina bifida occulta** may be signalled by a tuft of hair or a lipoma over the lumbar spine, or an incomplete dorsal vertebral arch may be noted on a lumbar spine X-ray. Severe forms produce large lumbosacral **myelomeningocoeles** (Fig. 31.1), which are visible at birth as fragile, weeping sacs on the lower back. The lower spinal cord has failed to develop, the legs are motionless, areflexic, and anaesthetic, and there is continual incontinence. Less severe forms spare the upper lumbar segments so that some proximal leg power is possible.

Without surgical repair, many babies die of meningitic infection through the spinal defect. Difficult ethical decisions surround the question of whether such repair should be attempted in severe cases of spina bifida where there is no prospect of useful leg function or sphincter control. Patients who survive the neonatal period are prone to hydrocephalus secondary to a Chiari malformation of the cerebellum which blocks drainage of cerebrospinal fluid (CSF) from the fourth ventricle (Fig. 31.2).

Obstructive hydrocephalus

Obstructive hydrocephalus simply means distension of the cerebral ventricles with cerebrospinal fluid which cannot drain freely. Brain scanning is diagnostic (see Fig. 7.8, p. 55). There are many causes, which include tumours of the cerebral hemisphere, pineal gland, brainstem, or cerebellum, all of which impede CSF flow. The form associated with a **Chiari malformation** of the cerebellar tonsils and spina bifida is mentioned above (Fig. 31.2). **Infantile hydrocephalus** produces a distinctively large head because the skull bone sutures do not fuse until the second year. Obstructive hydrocephalus is often due to cerebral aqueduct stenosis between the third and fourth ventricles, and the milder forms are often detected only in adulthood. Acute or severe hydrocephalus will cause headache, obvious loss of intellect, and may cause papilloedema. Milder hydrocephalus is more likely to cause gait uncertainty, a characteristic tendency to topple backwards, and urinary incontinence. Neurosurgical insertion of a ventriculo-peritoneal shunt releases the hydrocephalus, but can precipitate subdural haematomas if it allows too great a collapse of the cerebral ventricles.

CHAPTER 32

Psychologically determined symptoms

Chapter contents

Neurologists commonly see patients with symptoms or inconsistent physical signs which are not explicable by any recognized neurological disease. It is often clear that such symptoms or signs are being **manufactured psychologically**, be it consciously or unconsciously. Such patients are often polysymptomatic, and have a long history of consulting other specialists, particularly abdominal and gynaecological surgeons.

Various euphemisms and terms are used for these disorders, none of which is fully satisfactory: non-organic disease, medically unexplained symptoms, somatization, conversion disorder, and hysteria being commonest.

The **manner** in which such patients describe their symptoms may be discordant with the actual symptoms themselves. Relatively trivial symptoms such as tingling may be described in a vivid, florid, and exaggerated manner. Or a totally paralysed limb may be described in a smiling and unconcerned manner. Patients may be vague when asked about the time course. This difficult diagnostic area requires experience and even the most skilful diagnosticians get it wrong sometimes. Often the symptoms need full investigation before you can come to a definite conclusion that they originate psychologically. It is particularly difficult when psychologically determined symptoms occur in someone already suffering from a definite disease. Common examples include an exaggerated gait disorder in multiple sclerosis, pseudo-seizures in an epileptic, or exaggerated disability in an injured person seeking compensation.

It is likely that some patients currently considered to have 'non-organic' disorders will subsequently prove to be explicable in neurobiological terms. In the case of sensory symptoms, for example, the body is constantly receiving a barrage of afferent information, even when no discrete external stimulus is present. Normal perception involves positioning the threshold to a level below which such stimuli are considered normal and remain unnoticed. Abnormal interpretation of body state may involve erroneous positioning of this boundary to allow normal afferent information to be interpreted as abnormal.

Common psychologically determined symptoms include headache, facial pain, spinal pain, tinglings, patches of sensory loss, tunnel vision, tremor, blackouts, clumsiness, paralyses, memory blocks, dementia, and gait disorders.

Interpreting physical signs in patients with psychologically determined disorders

It is common to encounter patients with weakness or patterns of sensory disturbance that are wholly or partly determined psychologically. Although often bizarre, such physical signs should be calmly recorded as diagnostic phenomena. Care must be taken to avoid entering into a battle of wits with the patient.

Muscle power

The most characteristic feature is the **fluctuating** production of power by the muscles. Nonetheless the muscle can exert full power momentarily after encouragement. A muscle's strength may **collapse** after being normal for a moment. **Inconsistencies** in muscle power may be demonstrated. For instance, the patient may be unable to flex the hip against gravity on the couch, but will be observed to stand and flex the hip normally to put on trousers. The patient may have weakness of plantar flexion when tested on the couch, but be able to stand on tiptoe. Patients with psychologically determined weakness frequently accompany their unimpressive efforts with copious and theatrical grunting and sighing.

Sensation

Psychologically determined patches of sensory loss are often implausibly **sharply defined** with instantaneous transition from complete anaesthesia to normal sensation. It may be possible to demonstrate that these **boundaries shift** in position when the stimulus is presented at different speeds or from different directions,

particularly if the patient's eyes are shut. Sometimes you can demonstrate that the **numb limb changes sides** when the patient is rolled over and retested. Generally, psychologically determined patches of numbness do not obey the **anatomical territories** of peripheral nerves or nerve roots.

Gait disorders

Psychologically determined gait disorders are often **extremely athletic** or even balletic. For instance, patients may momentarily balance on one foot in midstride, which indicates extremely good motor control. Psychologically determined gaits usually **improve** when the patient thinks they are not being observed. Patients with psychologically determined gait disorders are often able to traverse an open space only to **fall theatrically** once they are able to grasp nearby furniture or an observer.

Psychopathology

In many patients, no detectable psychopathology underlies their psychologically determined symptoms. It must be stressed that psychological symptoms and signs are usually generated subconsciously.

Depression

Depression underlies many instances of tension headache, facial pain, and apparent dementia. You should ask specifically for the leading symptoms of melancholy, tearfulness, early wakening, weight fluctuation, and loss of interest in eating, sexual activity, hobbies, or family matters. Such patients often respond well to antidepressant drugs.

Anxiety states

Anxiety states may be responsible for tinglings, tremors, blackouts, or memory blocks. Sometimes these symptoms are due to hyperventilation. Typically, anxiety-provoked symptoms fluctuate markedly and may resolve for part of the day. For instance, the tingling of a true polyneuropathy does not disappear for half of the day. Reassurance that there is no serious disease, and teaching how to cope with hyperventilation are often effective. Some patients require benzodiazepines or psychotherapy.

Malingering

Malingering takes a number of forms. Not all are necessarily fully conscious; self-delusion can be prominent. Many are seeking compensation for alleged personal injury in road traffic accidents or at the hands of doctors. These usually feign a disabling symptom such as pain (which is difficult to disprove) or paralysis. A favourable court settlement may be the only cure. **Drug addicted** malingerers may feign intractable pain so as to obtain opiates. Mildly incapacitating symptoms can occur in the 'empty-nest syndrome', in which middle-aged women seemingly wish to tie their husbands into the home at a time when their children are leaving.

Conversion hysteria

True conversion hysteria is uncommon. Such patients seem to accept quite placidly that their paralysis or gait disorder is an incurable condition. Many are female and frequently have a long history of gynaecological and sexual symptoms, and surgical operations. Sometimes the history will disclose a similar paralysis in a parent, which has acted as a template. Such patients can be permanently wheelchair bound, and no treatment seems to help.

Treating psychologically determined symptoms

Should you confront patients with your diagnosis that their symptoms are psychologically determined? If you are blunt in doing so, the patient will dig in so as not to lose face, may denounce you as a hopeless doctor and seek another with whom to repeat the whole performance, or they may generate a new and different batch of symptoms. It is usually more productive to reassure the patient that you have been unable to detect any serious disease to explain their symptoms, and stress that this is encouraging since it means that the symptoms are likely to resolve spontaneously over the next few days or weeks. Frank lies, such as blaming a virus infection, are best avoided. Bluntly telling patients that you think that depression or anxiety are the root cause of their symptoms is likely to raise hackles and prevent compliance with any medication you prescribe. It is usually better to say 'I think your original symptoms have led to a bit of secondary anxiety and depression, which has set up a vicious circle which is making those original symptoms much more noticeable. If we can break that vicious circle by treating the depressive component, it will probably allow your underlying symptoms to get completely better.' Some patients with severe symptoms due to psychological factors will require expert psychiatric help. Behavioural approaches involve setting objectives for overcoming certain disabling symptoms.

CASE 32.1 'IT WASN'T MY BODY'

A woman in her 30s developed complete paraplegia one morning but seemed rather vague about whether this had come on instantaneously or whether it had evolved over hours. Bladder control and leg sensation remained normal. The admitting doctors fully expected to find an areflexic paraparesis typical of early Guillain–Barré syndrome, or the extensor plantars and sensory level typical of acute spinal cord disease, such as myelitis. However, they were surprised to find no abnormalities apart from otherwise normal legs that simply didn't move. MRI confirmed that there was no intrinsic or extrinsic lesion affecting the spinal cord, the spinal fluid was normal, and nerve conduction studies revealed no polyneuropathy. Suspecting that the weakness was psychologically determined, the patient was reassured, and rehabilitated. Within a day fluctuating levels of voluntary power returned to the legs, which would often collapse dramatically after initially exerting normal power. A few days later she walked out of hospital quite normally. Her doctors had explored gently whether there was any reason for this acute psychologically determined paraparesis, but unrevealingly. Just before leaving hospital the patient confided in a physiotherapist that at a party during the night before becoming paralysed she had found herself in bed with someone other than her long-standing boyfriend. She did not wish any follow up.

Comment

- As is often the case, we never discovered to what extent the processes causing this psychologically determined paralysis were conscious. We interpreted her disorder as a form of denial of the lower half of her body which in turn had acted as the physical focus for unwelcome emotions.

- Although neurologists encounter psychologically determined muscle weakness quite frequently, it is most unusual to identify a discrete precipitating psychosocial event, such as this.

- It is characteristic of such patients that they are vague about the timing, and speed of onset of their weakness or other symptoms. Inconsistencies and fluctuations are usually evident on testing. And of course no unequivocally abnormal physical signs, such as extensor plantars, are present.

Index

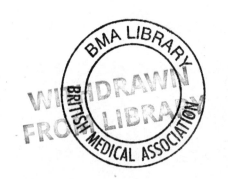